TOP TRAILS™

Shenandoah National Park

MUST-DO HIKES FOR EVERYONE

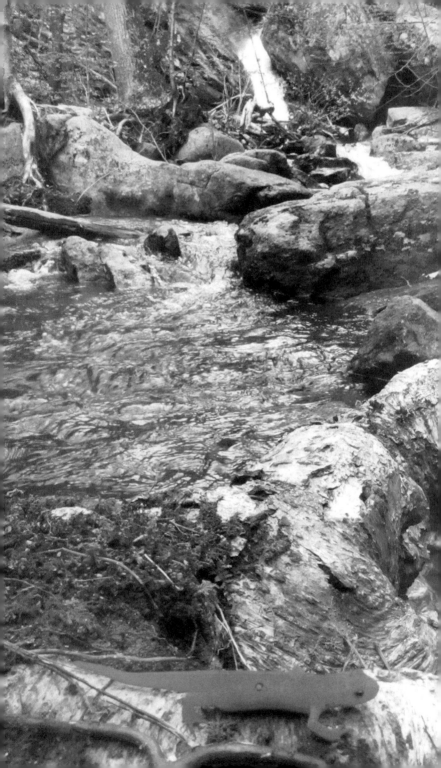

TOP TRAILS™

Shenandoah National Park

MUST-DO HIKES FOR EVERYONE

Written by

Johnny Molloy

🐾 **WILDERNESS PRESS** ... *on the trail since 1967*

Top Trails Shenandoah National Park: Must-Do Hikes for Everyone

1st EDITION 2012

Copyright © 2012 by Johnny Molloy
Front cover photo copyright © 2012 by Johnny Molloy
Interior photos, except where noted, by the author
Maps and elevation profiles: Johnny Molloy and Scott McGrew
Cover design: Frances Baca Design and Scott McGrew
Interior design: Frances Baca Design
Layout: Amber Kaye Henderson
Editor: Laura Shauger
Index: Rich Carlson

ISBN 978-0-89997-679-2
Manufactured in the United States of America

Published by: **Wilderness Press**
               Keen Communications
               PO Box 43673
               Birmingham, AL 35243
               (800) 443-7227
               info@wildernesspress.com
               www.wildernesspress.com

Visit our website for a complete listing of our books and for ordering information.
Distributed by Publishers Group West

Cover photo: View from Hawksbill (Trail 25)
Frontispiece: Salamander in repose on Hazel River (Trail 16)

The Top Trails™ Series

Wilderness Press

When Wilderness Press published *Sierra North* in 1967, no other trail guide like it existed for the Sierra backcountry. The first run of 2,800 copies sold out in less than two months and its success heralded the beginning of Wilderness Press. Since we were founded more than 40 years ago, we have expanded our territories to cover California, Alaska, Hawaii, the U.S. Southwest, the Pacific Northwest, New England, Canada, and the Southeast.

Wilderness Press continues to publish comprehensive, accurate, and readable outdoor books. Hikers, backpackers, kayakers, skiers, snowshoers, climbers, cyclists, and trail runners rely on Wilderness Press for accurate outdoor adventure information.

Top Trails

In its Top Trails guides, Wilderness Press has paid special attention to organization so that you can find the perfect hike each and every time. Whether you're looking for a steep trail to test yourself on or a walk in the park, a romantic waterfall, or a city view, Top Trails will lead you there.

Each Top Trails guide contains trails for everyone. The trails selected provide a sampling of the best that the region has to offer. These are the must-do hikes, walks, runs, and bike rides, with every feature of the area represented.

Every book in the Top Trails series offers:

- The Wilderness Press commitment to accuracy and reliability
- Ratings and rankings for each trail
- Distances and approximate times
- Easy-to-follow trail notes
- Map and permit information

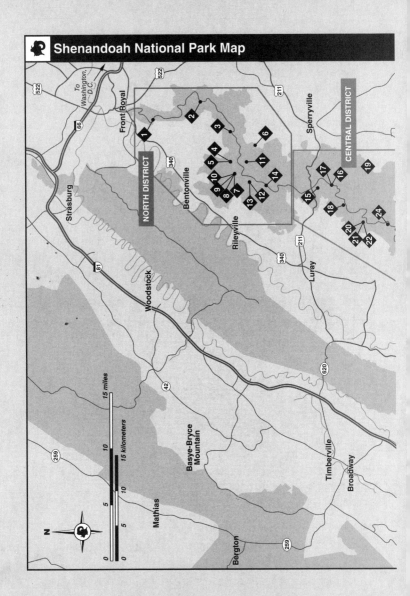

Shenandoah National Park Map

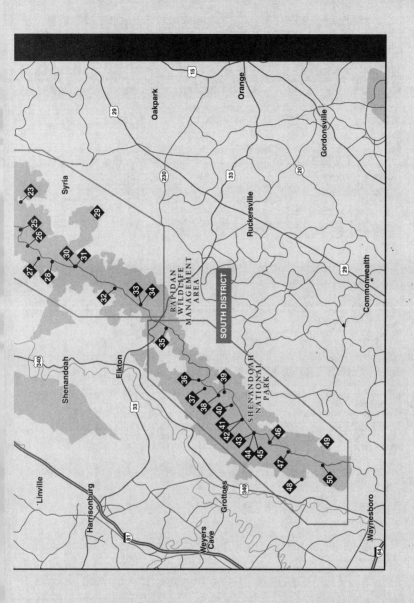

Shenandoah National Park Trails

TRAIL NUMBER AND NAME	Page	Difficulty -12345+	Length in Miles	Type	Backpacking	Dayhiking	Child-Friendly	Pets Prohibited
1. North District								
1 Dickey Ridge Historic Hike	27	2	4.3	Loop		Dayhiking		Pets Prohibited
2 Compton Peak	33	3	3.2	Out & Back		Dayhiking		
3 Big Devils Stairs Vista	37	3	5.0	Out & Back	Backpacking	Dayhiking		
4 Sugarloaf Loop	43	3	4.7	Loop	Backpacking	Dayhiking		
5 Overall Run Falls	49	4	6.8	Out & Back		Dayhiking		
6 Little Devils Stairs Loop	55	4	5.4	Loop	Backpacking	Dayhiking		
7 Traces Nature Trail	61	2	1.6	Loop		Dayhiking	Child-Friendly	Pets Prohibited
8 Overall Run Loop	67	5	9.2	Loop	Backpacking	Dayhiking		
9 Heiskell Hollow Loop	73	4	7.2	Loop	Backpacking	Dayhiking		
10 Elkwallow Loop	77	3	5.6	Loop		Dayhiking		
11 Piney River Falls	83	4	6.8	Out & Back	Backpacking	Dayhiking		
12 Knob Mountain and Jeremys Run Loop	89	5	13.1	Loop	Backpacking	Dayhiking		
13 Neighbor Mountain and Jeremys Run Loop	95	5	14.0	Loop	Backpacking	Dayhiking		
14 Thornton River Loop	101	4	7.9	Loop	Backpacking	Dayhiking		
2. Central District								
15 Marys Rock via The Pinnacle	121	3	7.2	Out & Back		Dayhiking		
16 Hazel Falls and Cave	127	3	5.2	Out & Back		Dayhiking	Child-Friendly	
17 Hazel Country Loop	131	4	7.9	Loop	Backpacking	Dayhiking		
18 Corbin Cabin Hike	135	3	2.8	Out & Back		Dayhiking		
19 Old Rag Loop	139	5	9.1	Loop		Dayhiking		Pets Prohibited
20 Stony Man Loop	145	3	3.4	Loop		Dayhiking		Pets Prohibited
21 Robertson Mountain	151	4	6.8	Out & Back		Dayhiking		
22 Millers Head	157	2	1.4	Out & Back		Dayhiking	Child-Friendly	
23 Falls of Whiteoak Canyon	163	4	5.2	Out & Back		Dayhiking		
24 Cedar Run Falls	169	4	3.4	Out & Back		Dayhiking		
25 Hawksbill Summit	175	2	2.2	Out & Back		Dayhiking		

TYPE
- Loop
- Out & Back

DIFFICULTY
- 1 2 3 4 5 +
less   more

USES & ACCESS
- Dayhiking
- Backpacking
- Child-Friendly
- Pets Prohibited

TERRAIN
- Summit
- Ridgeline
- Stream
- Waterfall

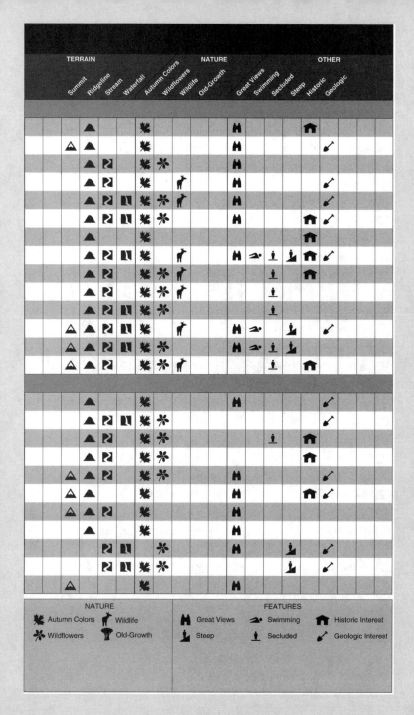

NATURE — Autumn Colors, Wildflowers, Wildlife, Old-Growth

FEATURES — Great Views, Swimming, Historic Interest, Steep, Secluded, Geologic Interest

Shenandoah National Park Trails

TRAIL NUMBER AND NAME	Page	Difficulty -12345+	Length in Miles	Type	Backpacking	Dayhiking	Child-Friendly	Pets Prohibited
2. Central District (continued)								
26 Rose River Falls Loop	179	3	4.0	Loop	Backpacking	Dayhiking		
27 Lewis Spring Falls Loop	185	3	3.3	Loop		Dayhiking		
28 Hazeltop and Rapidan Camp Loop	191	4	7.2	Loop	Backpacking	Dayhiking		
29 Bear Church Rock via Staunton River	197	5	7.6	Out & Back	Backpacking	Dayhiking		
30 Bear Church Rock from Bootens Gap	201	4	9.4	Out & Back		Dayhiking		
31 Conway River Loop	205	5	12.0	Loop	Backpacking	Dayhiking		Pets Prohibited
32 Pocosin Mission	213	2	2.0	Out & Back		Dayhiking	Child-Friendly	
33 South River Falls Loop	219	3	4.5	Loop		Dayhiking		
34 Saddleback Mountain Loop	225	2	3.9	Loop		Dayhiking	Child-Friendly	
3. South District								
35 Hightop	243	3	3.2	Out & Back	Backpacking	Dayhiking		
36 Rocky Mount Loop	247	5	9.8	Loop	Backpacking	Dayhiking		
37 Rocky Mountain Loop	253	5	9.5	Loop	Backpacking	Dayhiking		
38 Loft Mountain Loop	259	2	2.9	Loop		Dayhiking		Pets Prohibited
39 Patterson Ridge Loop	265	5	9.7	Loop	Backpacking	Dayhiking		
40 Big Run Loop	271	3	5.8	Loop		Dayhiking		
41 Rockytop and Big Run Loop	277	5	13.3	Loop	Backpacking	Dayhiking		
42 Austin Mountain and Madison Run Loop	283	4	8.8	Loop	Backpacking	Dayhiking		
43 Falls Loop from Browns Gap	289	4	7.0	Loop	Backpacking	Dayhiking		
44 Furnace Mountain via Blackrock	295	3	6.8	Out & Back	Backpacking	Dayhiking		
45 Blackrock Loop	301	1	1.1	Loop		Dayhiking	Child-Friendly	
46 Big Branch Falls via Moormans River	305	4	7.6	Out & Back	Backpacking	Dayhiking		
47 Chimney Rock	309	2	3.2	Out & Back	Backpacking	Dayhiking		
48 Chimney Rock via Riprap Hollow	315	4	6.8	Out & Back		Dayhiking		
49 Turk Mountain	321	2	2.4	Out & Back		Dayhiking		
50 Turk Branch Loop	325	4	7.5	Loop	Backpacking	Dayhiking		

TYPE	USES & ACCESS	TERRAIN
Loop	Dayhiking Child-Friendly	Summit Stream
Out & Back	Backpacking Pets Prohibited	Ridgeline Waterfall
DIFFICULTY - 1 2 3 4 5 + less more		

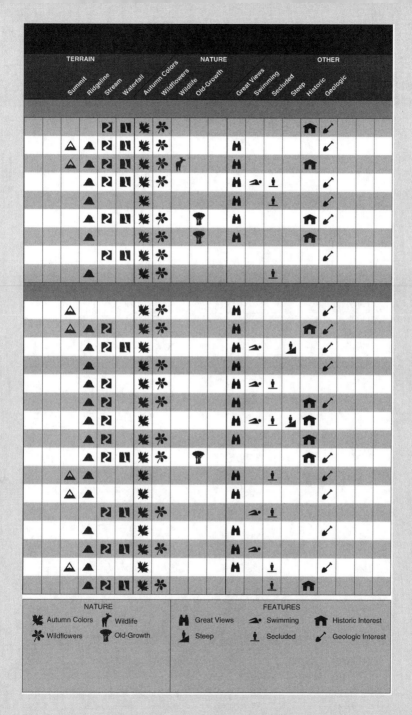

Contents

Shenandoah National Park Map vi
Shenandoah National Park Trails Table viii

Using Top Trails xvi
   Organization of Top Trails xvi
   Choosing a Trail. xix

Introduction to Shenandoah National Park. 1
   Geography and Topography. 3
   Flora. 4
   Fauna 5
   When to Go 6
   Weather and Seasons 7
   Trail Selection 8
   Key Features. 8
   Multiple Uses 8

On the Trail 9
   Have a Plan 9
   Carry the Essentials 10
   Useful But Less than Essential Items. 11
   Trail Etiquette 12

CHAPTER 1
North District 15

  1 Dickey Ridge Historic Hike. 27
  2 Compton Peak 33
  3 Big Devils Stairs Vista 37
  4 Sugarloaf Loop 43
  5 Overall Run Falls 49
  6 Little Devils Stairs Loop 55
  7 Traces Nature Trail 61
  8 Overall Run Loop 67
  9 Heiskell Hollow Loop 73

10 Elkwallow Loop 77
11 Piney River Falls 83
12 Knob Mountain and Jeremys Run Loop 89
13 Neighbor Mountain and Jeremys Run Loop 95
14 Thornton River Loop 101

CHAPTER 2
Central District 107

15 Marys Rock via The Pinnacle 121
16 Hazel Falls and Cave 127
17 Hazel Country Loop 131
18 Corbin Cabin Hike 135
19 Old Rag Loop 139
20 Stony Man Loop 145
21 Robertson Mountain 151
22 Millers Head 157
23 Falls of Whiteoak Canyon 163
24 Cedar Run Falls 169
25 Hawksbill Summit 175
26 Rose River Falls Loop 179
27 Lewis Spring Falls Loop 185
28 Hazeltop and Rapidan Camp Loop 191
29 Bear Church Rock via Staunton River 197
30 Bear Church Rock from Bootens Gap 201
31 Conway River Loop 205
32 Pocosin Mission 213
33 South River Falls Loop 219
34 Saddleback Mountain Loop 225

CHAPTER 3
South District 229

35 Hightop. 243
36 Rocky Mount Loop 247
37 Rocky Mountain Loop 253
38 Loft Mountain Loop 259
39 Patterson Ridge Loop 265
40 Big Run Loop 271
41 Rockytop and Big Run Loop 277
42 Austin Mountain and Madison Run Loop 283
43 Falls Loop from Browns Gap 289

44 Furnace Mountain via Blackrock 295
45 Blackrock Loop 301
46 Big Branch Falls via Moormans River 305
47 Chimney Rock 309
48 Chimney Rock via Riprap Hollow 315
49 Turk Mountain 321
50 Turk Branch Loop 325

Appendix: Local Resources................................. 330
Index 332

About the Author 338

Using Top Trails™

Organization of Top Trails

Top Trails is designed to make identifying the perfect trail easy and enjoyable, and to make every outing a success and a pleasure. With this book you'll find it's a snap to find the right trail, whether you're planning a major hike or just a sociable stroll with friends.

The Region

Each Top Trails begins with the regional map (pages vi–vii), displaying the entire area covered by the guide and providing an overview of the geography. The map is clearly marked to show which area is covered by each chapter.

After the regional map comes the master trails table (pages viii–xi), which lists every trail covered in the guide. Here you'll find a concise description, basic information, and highlighted features, all indispensable when planning an outing. A quick reading of the regional map and trails table will give you a good overview of the entire region covered by the book.

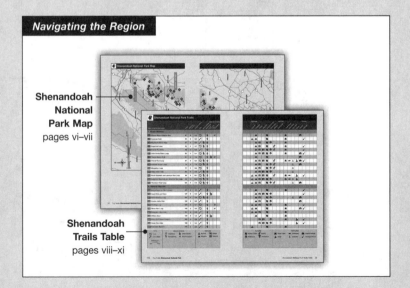

Navigating the Region

Shenandoah National Park Map pages vi–vii

Shenandoah Trails Table pages viii–xi

The Areas

The region covered in each book is divided into areas, with each chapter corresponding to one area in the region. Each area chapter introduction starts with information to help you choose and enjoy a trail every time out. Use the table of contents or the regional map to identify an area of interest, and then turn to the area chapter to find the following:

- An overview of the area, including park and permit information
- An area map showing all trail locations
- A trail features table providing trail-by-trail details
- Trail summaries highlighting each trail's specific features

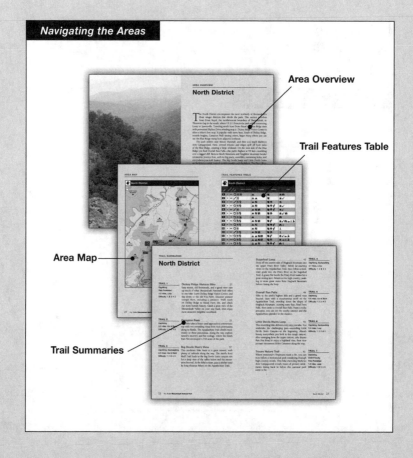

Navigating the Areas

Area Overview

Trail Features Table

Area Map

Trail Summaries

The Trails

The basic building block of the Top Trails guide is the trail entry. Each one is laid out to make finding and following the trail as simple as possible, with all pertinent information presented in this easy-to-follow format:

- A detailed trail map
- Trail descriptors covering difficulty, length, and other essential data
- A written trail description
- Trail milestones providing easy-to-follow, turn-by-turn trail directions

Some trail descriptions offer additional information:

- An elevation profile
- Trail options
- Trail highlights

In the margins of the trail entries, keep your eyes open for graphic icons that signal features mentioned in the text.

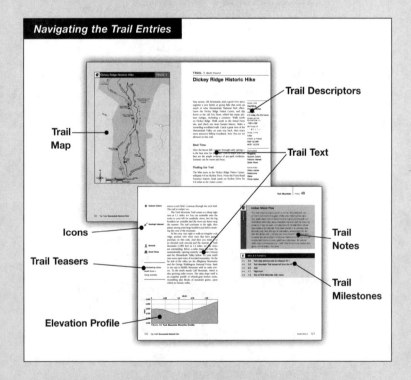

Navigating the Trail Entries

Trail Map · Trail Descriptors · Trail Text · Icons · Trail Teasers · Elevation Profile · Trail Notes · Trail Milestones

Choosing a Trail

Top Trails provides several different ways of choosing a trail, all presented in easy-to-read tables, charts, and maps.

Location

If you know in general where you want to go, Top Trails makes it easy to find the right trail in the right place. Each chapter begins with a large-scale map showing the starting point of every trail in that area.

Features

This guide describes the Top Trails of Shenandoah National Park, and each trail is chosen because it offers one or more features that make it appealing. Using the trail descriptors, summaries, and tables, you can quickly examine all the trails for the features they offer or seek a particular feature among the list of trails.

Best Time

Time of year and current conditions can be important factors in selecting the best trail. For example, an exposed low-elevation trail may be a riot of color in early spring, but an oven-baked taste of hell in midsummer. Wherever relevant, Top Trails identifies the best and worst conditions for the trails you plan to hike.

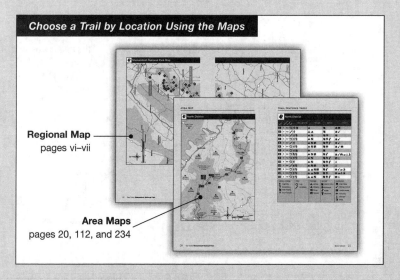

Choose a Trail by Location Using the Maps

Regional Map — pages vi–vii

Area Maps pages 20, 112, and 234

Difficulty

Every trail has an overall difficulty rating on a scale of 1 to 5, which takes into consideration length, elevation change, exposure, trail quality, etc., to create one (admittedly subjective) rating.

The ratings assume you are an able-bodied adult in reasonably good shape, using the trail for hiking. The ratings also assume normal weather conditions—clear and dry.

Readers should make an honest assessment of their own abilities and adjust time estimates accordingly. Also, rain, snow, heat, wind, and poor visibility can all affect your pace on even the easiest of trails.

The Elevation Factor

Cumulative Elevation Gain and Loss

The at-a-glance info shown in the margin of each Top Trails entry includes a pair of numbers labeled Cumulative Elevation +/-. The numbers represent the *total gain* and/or *total loss of altitude* as you negotiate the trail's ascents and descents between the beginning and ending points of the hike.

For hikes that start and end at the same spot—i.e., a loop or an out-and-back trail—the elevation gain matches the elevation loss because you are essentially retracing your route. (Exceptions may occur—and are reflected in

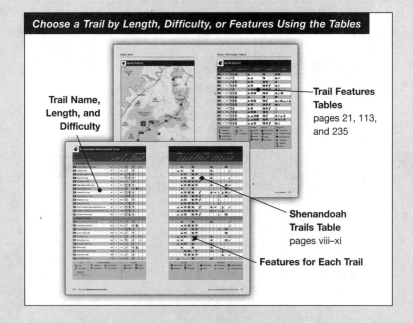

Choose a Trail by Length, Difficulty, or Features Using the Tables

Trail Name, Length, and Difficulty

Trail Features Tables
pages 21, 113, and 235

Shenandoah Trails Table
pages viii–xi

Features for Each Trail

Map Legend

Featured trail	————————		
Alternate trail	- - - - - - - -		
Appalachian Trail	– – –◇– – –		
Interstate	══⟨40⟩⟨440⟩══	Water body	
Major road	—⟨9⟩⟨28A⟩—	River/creek	
Minor road	—⟨614⟩—	Intermittent stream	
Unpaved road	═══════	Park boundary	

Amphitheatre	♨	Radio tower	⌶
Campground/campsite	▲	Rapids/cascades	⌇
Cemetery	✝	Ranger station	♠
Equestrian trail	🐎	Restroom	♀♂
Gate	⚲	Shelter	⊏
Marsh area	⋟	Spring	○
Milepost	12/4	Swimming access	🏊
Mine site	⚔	Tower	員
Parking area	🅿	Trailhead and parking	🚶
Peak	▲	Vista point	Ħ
Picnic area	🎋	Waterfall	∥
Point of interest	●		

Top Trails Difficulty Ratings

1 A short trail, generally level, that can be completed in one hour or less.

2 A route of 1 to 3 miles, with some up and down, that can be completed in one to two hours.

3 A longer route, up to 5 miles, with uphill and/or downhill sections.

4 A long or steep route, perhaps more than 5 miles, or with climbs of more than 1,000 vertical feet.

5 The most severe route, both long and steep, more than 5 miles long with climbs of more than 1,000 vertical feet.

the numbers—if the author includes, for example, an optional spur that you take outbound but not inbound.) With a point-to-point route, the gain and loss will most likely differ. In either case, for matching or differing figures, the author provides both sets of numbers, preceded by a plus or minus sign.

Example: Picture an out-and-back trail that starts at 1,500', climbs to 1,700', descends to 1,500', and climbs to 2,800' at the turnaround point. The hiker reverses course and descends 1,300', climbs 200', and descends 200'. Coming and going, the elevation gain totals 1,300', and the elevation loss totals 1,300'. This would be represented as cumulative elevation: +1,300'/-1,300' for this hike.

But what if at that 2,800' point, the hiker has arranged for a shuttle, and this is a point-to-point hike? The cumulative elevation change would be +1,500'/-200'.

Elevation Profile

To illustrate those incremental ups and downs, each Top Trails entry includes an elevation profile. This illustration graphically portrays the rises and falls you can expect along the hike. For example, one trail's cumulative elevation may total +1,300'/-1,300', and the elevation profile shows that the gain and loss occur as you climb and descend only one peak. Another trail's cumulative elevation may be identical: +1,300'/-1,300'. However its elevation profile may show that you will have many small rises and falls all along the trail to reach that total.

Thus, you will want to review both the cumulative elevation number(s) *and* the elevation profile to know whether your climbs and descents will be many small ones or a few long and arduous ones.

Introduction to Shenandoah National Park

Shenandoah National Park is a scenic mountain haven of the eastern seaboard, a glittering jewel in the Appalachian range. What makes Shenandoah so special? First, consider panoramic views from overlooks scattered along lofty Skyline Drive, which runs the length of the 300-square-mile sanctuary. Beyond Skyline Drive lies another Shenandoah, where bears furtively roam the hollows and brook trout ply the tumbling streams. Quartz, granite, and greenstone outcrops jut above the diverse forest, allowing far-flung views of the Blue Ridge and surrounding Shenandoah Valley.

You must reach this other Shenandoah, beyond Skyline Drive, by foot. The rewards increase with every footfall beneath the stately oaks of the ridgetops and in the deep canyons where waterfalls roar among old-growth trees spared by the logger's axe. In some places your footsteps lead past what once were pioneer farms. These homesites reveal another era of Shenandoah. This rich cultural history once found settlers squeezed into the narrow valleys and apple orchards lining grassy fields atop the ridges, where lives were made in the craggy Appalachian highlands.

This meld of natural and cultural history is fitting in Virginia, where so much of this country's story has been played out, from the battles of the American Revolution and Civil War to battles in Congress where this park was established. Shenandoah National Park has also seen the cutting down and reforestation of the park, the building of Skyline Drive, the return of the deer and bear, and the invasion of exotic pests that threaten the mountain trees. It has seen park facilities built, fall to disrepair, and become new again. And through it all, Shenandoah has shone.

Shenandoah National Park continues to undergo changes. And in nature, changes come quickly and slowly—quickly as in the human-caused Smith Run Fire of 2011, the prescribed burns to preserve Big Meadows, or the thousand-year flood of 1995. But changes also come slowly, such as the recovery from the gypsy moth infestation of the 1990s and the demise of the hemlock from the hemlock woolly adelgid in the early 2000s. But Shenandoah continues to display its mountain beauty and come back better than ever. Air quality continues to improve since a low point in the 1970s, allowing for more extensive views year-round.

Choosing Shenandoah as a place to spend your free time is a wise decision. And yet the park can be intimidating, especially for the first-time visitor. Not only are there hundreds of miles of trails running like veins down and along a narrow mountain spine, but with millions of guests annually, Shenandoah National Park is a heavily visited destination—quite intimidating indeed. This book was conceived to make the backcountry majesty of Shenandoah more accessible to visitors.

With this national park's many trails and people, discovering its beauty and solitude can be a hit-or-miss proposition. Where are the spectacular vistas? Where are the waterfalls and the old settlers' homesites? Where can I find solitude? Leaving it all to chance doesn't offer good odds for an all-too-brief vacation from the rat race. Weeks spent daydreaming of a fleeting slice of freedom could culminate in a three-hour driving marathon or a noisy walk up a crowded trail. Fortunately, with this book and a little bit of planning and forethought, you can make the most of your national park experience.

May this book be as beneficial to your Shenandoah experience as it has been to mine. I have been hiking Shenandoah since the 1980s and have had a Shenandoah guide in print since 1998, with multiple updated and improved editions. Penning this guide for Wilderness Press gave me the chance to rehike all the trails and write another guide to what I think is one of the most beautiful places in the United States. You will find this very accessible guide a marked improvement over my previous ones to the park.

This book presents a variety of hikes. The majority steer you toward the most scenic areas, giving you the opportunity to enjoy your time on the trail instead of behind someone else's car. Most hikes seek solitude to maximize your Shenandoah experience. However, as the subtitle suggests, there are some must-do popular hikes. Consequently, a few hikes traverse popular and potentially crowded areas. Each hike lists a "best time" that will help you manage the trails to your advantage.

This book presents 50 hikes. Classic hikes, such as Old Rag and the falls of Whiteoak Canyon, and seldom-visited gems, such as Piney River Falls and Furnace Mountain, are all included. Though the latter are not as well known, they offer more solitude than and equally scenic sights as the more popular hikes so that you can discover Shenandoah on your own terms.

Often, park sightseers pick a hike randomly without knowing where it will lead, or they follow the crowds wherever they go. Many times, I've been stopped with the question, "What's down this trail?" Choosing a hike at random in Shenandoah, where many trails drop steeply off the Blue Ridge, may result in a disappointing trip followed by a rigorous return to the car with little reward to show for your effort. This guide provides easy means to find hikes to suit your desires.

Two types of hikes are offered: one-way and loop hikes. One-way hikes lead to a particularly rewarding destination and return via the same trail. The return trip allows you to see everything from the opposite vantage point. You may notice more minute trailside features the second go-round. Returning at a different time of day may give the same trail a surprisingly different character. But to some, returning on the same trail simply isn't enjoyable. Some hikers can't stand the thought of covering the same ground twice with 500 other miles of Shenandoah trails awaiting them. The loop hikes provide an alternative.

Dayhiking is the best and most popular way to break into the Shenandoah wilderness. But for those with the inclination to see the mountain cycle from day to night and back again can enjoy many of these hikes too. Backpackers must follow park backcountry camping regulations and practice "leave no trace" wilderness-use etiquette. Backpackers can capture the changing moods of the mountains as day turns to night, the weather cycles with the sun, and the permanent park residents go about their business of surviving and reproducing.

When touring Shenandoah, it's tempting to remain in your car and enjoy the sights along Skyline Drive. While auto touring allows an overview of the park, vehicles create a barrier between you and the wilderness beyond. Windshield tourists hoping to observe wildlife often end up observing only the cars around them. While overlooks avail easy views, the hassle of driving, the drone of the car engine, and the lack of effort in reaching the views can make them less than inspirational. Shenandoah is great for hiking.

The wilderness experience can unleash your mind and body, allowing you to relax and find peace and quiet. It also enables you to grasp beauty and splendor: a white-quartz outcrop with a window overlooking the patchwork valley below, a bobcat disappearing into a laurel thicket, or a snow-covered clearing marking an old homestead. On these protected lands you can let your mind roam where it pleases—something you simply can't achieve in a climate-controlled automobile. Hiking is the best way to enjoy this special preserve; get out and enjoy Shenandoah.

Geography and Topography

The topography of Shenandoah results from the weathering of one of the oldest mountain ranges in the world—the Appalachians. Shenandoah National Park overlays a long stretch of the Blue Ridge, whose billion-year-old rocks rise above the forest. The main spine of the park stretches for 70 miles end to end, dividing the bucolic Shenandoah Valley from the

Piedmont to the east. Elevations vary from 4,050 feet atop Hawksbill down to less than 550 feet near Front Royal. This vertical variation is one of the reasons for the incredible diversity of life found within its boundaries.

Shenandoah National Park forms the headwaters to many a stream flowing west and east from the north-south oriented Blue Ridge. The South Fork Shenandoah River system absorbs all waterways spilling west from the park. The South Fork meets the North Fork Shenandoah River just north of the park, melding their waters and contributing them to the Potomac River, which in turn flows through the District of Columbia to the sea. The streams draining to the east are a little more complicated. Tributaries of the Rivanna River, including Doyles River and Moormans River, flow from the mountains of the South District to meet the James River, flowing through Richmond to the sea. In the Central District, the Rapidan River and its tributaries from the South River to Thornton River find their way to the Piedmont and the Rappahannock River, which flows through Fredericksburg, pushing into Chesapeake Bay. In the North District, smaller streams also course east into the headwaters of the Rappahannock and beyond.

The dominant landform is the high, continuous ridge extending north-south from one end of Shenandoah to the other—the Blue Ridge. In addition to dividing river drainages, it also forms the boundary for numerous Old Dominion counties. Often-rocky shoulder ridges, like ribs protruding from a backbone, extend from the Blue Ridge and separate steep, yet deeply wooded valleys cut by eons of precipitation.

Flora

Shenandoah harbors plant species from throughout the Appalachian chain, from the hardwoods of the South to evergreens normally found in boreal climes, clinging to the highest points. Of course, the trees are the most visible piece of these complex ecosystems, gently overlapping and intermingling. Below the canopy rises more life. The Shenandoah you see today is the result of park protection, for much of this preserve was razed and used as pasture. There are few old-growth stands of trees; however, sporadic old-growth giants can be found along many trails. But the native ecosystems have reclaimed their rightful spots on the mountains. It is not just the showy trees and wildflowers blooming throughout the warm season that get attention; Shenandoah also has amazing arrays of humble yet biologically important plants from mosses to fungi.

This diverse plant mosaic blends and divides depending on elevation, precipitation, and exposure. But the great oak forests of Shenandoah are a starting point. Growing along the ridges and slopes of the mountains, red and chestnut oaks stand sturdy while producing fall mast for wildlife. Mountain laurel, dogwood, and scraggly pines often accompany the great oaks. In the park's lower reaches grow Southern temperate woodlands, an agglomeration of hardwoods from sourwood to sassafras in drier areas. Cove hardwoods tower over lower reaches in hollows, dominated by tulip trees. Along the streams towering white pines, black birch, and mountain laurel provide shade. The hemlocks have been decimated by the hemlock woolly adelgid. Some stands and individual trees have been preserved and hopefully will regenerate in the future.

On the higher ridges with cooler, moister conditions and the highest elevation watersheds, the vegetation morphs into northern hardwoods, such as yellow birch, beech, and cherry. Rise still higher and you will occasionally find red spruce or Fraser fir trees, the two northern climate trees that hug the highest peaks of the Appalachians, where it is still cool enough for them to survive. Shenandoah has no great stretches of boreal forest, just small pockets of trees sprinkled in the highlands. Throughout the park, locust, pine, and brambles are reclaiming former clearings, transforming them into towering woodlands once again. Together these forest types, blending and intermingling, comprise a diverse biological ecosystem worthy of national park protection.

Fauna

The Shenandoah's rich vegetational environment and large wildlands support an impressive array of mammals—more than 50 species. The black bear roams throughout Shenandoah. From the rich acorn crops of the oak forests to the fruit trees from pioneer homesteads to berries growing rampant in former fields, bears have a wide variety of food sources within the park. Don't be surprised if you see a bruin in this park. There is no doubt you will see white-tailed deer. When the park was populated by pioneers, unregulated hunting nearly drove the deer from Shenandoah, but today they are found along Skyline Drive and beyond. Drivers must constantly look out for these gentle creatures. They can also be found in the woods and especially in historically cleared areas such as Big Meadows.

A quiet hiker may also witness turkeys on wooded hillsides or in clearings. Furtive bobcats can sometimes be spotted crossing trails. Raccoons are occasionally seen in the wild. Coyotes are found throughout the park but will usually spot you before you see them. A bounding tan tail disappearing into the distance will likely comprise a sighting of this critter, which effectively replaced the extirpated red wolf in the East.

Extensive efforts have been made to keep all animals wild in Shenandoah. Gone are the days of roadside feedings. Education and bearproof garbage cans have reduced negative interactions between people and wildlife.

More than 200 birds either live in the park or migrate through it. These avians, including pileated woodpeckers and red-tailed hawks, ply the forest for food. The eastern screech owl emits a goose bump–raising call. Songbirds native to the north and south find a home in the park.

Shenandoah's north-south orientation adds to its importance as a migratory bird corridor. Birding is a popular pastime in the park and can add to any hike.

The park's waters harbor about three dozen types of fish. Most famously, Shenandoah is a bastion for brook trout. Unlike the Smokies, this park never had rainbow or brook trout intentionally introduced into its waters. "Brookies" are the

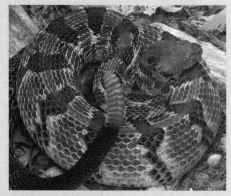

Rattlesnakes *may be encountered on the trail—especially in sunny, rocky areas.*

only native to Shenandoah. Technically, the brook is not a true trout, but a char. Brooks prefer cold clear waters and are found in more than 50 of the park's 90 streams. Brown trout have been making their way into the lower reaches of Shenandoah's streams, and biologists are trying to limit their numbers.

Spend some time hiking at Shenandoah, and you may be surprised by the variety of snakes in the area, 18 in all. Most encounters will be with non-venomous specimens. However, two poisonous snakes—copperhead and timber rattler—call the park home. Copperheads can be found near streams and on outcrops, whereas rattlers will primarily be seen sunning on rocks. Shenandoah harbors 14 types of salamanders, including the rare Shenandoah salamander, found only within the park. It is just one more example of how the life in these mountains lives up to its national park status.

When to Go

Shenandoah has a somewhat undeserved reputation of being overcrowded. Yes, Skyline Drive and its overlooks and facilities can be crowded during summer, on warm season weekends, and on holidays. The roads can also be busy during the October leaf-viewing season. However, get a quarter mile from a trailhead on 95 percent of the hiking trails, and you will experience solitude. Busy trails—and there are some—are noted in the trail descriptions.

Shenandoah National Park is a four-season destination. Hikers with well-thought-out plans can easily execute their treks beyond the obvious busy times. Try to hike midweek and just before or after major holidays. Spring is a great time, with its renewing vibrancy exemplified by colorful wildflowers and budding trees. Fall can be rewarding too, but avoid October weekends. Solitude can be found anytime during winter. As far as busy trails go, try to hike them early in the morning or later in the evening. Iffy weather—50 percent or more chance of rain—often keeps the crowds away. If you can, avoid busy trails on nice weather weekends.

Weather and Seasons

Each of the four distinct seasons lays its hands on Shenandoah National Park, though elevation always factors into park weather patterns. While each season brings exciting changes in the flora and fauna, the changes can occur seemingly day to day rather than month to month.

Be prepared for a wide range of temperatures and conditions regardless of the season. As a rule of thumb, the temperature decreases about three degrees for every 1,000 feet of elevation gained. The approximately 50 inches of yearly precipitation on the Blue Ridge is about 15 inches more than the nearby Shenandoah Valley receives. This precipitation is evenly distributed throughout the year, though it arrives with slow-moving frontal systems in winter and with thunderstorms in summer.

The chart below is from Luray, Virginia, located in the Shenandoah Valley, just west of the park. Expect temperatures in the higher park elevations to be 10 degrees cooler.

Average High and Low Temperature (°F) by Month, Luray, Virginia						
	JAN	FEB	MARCH	APRIL	MAY	JUNE
High	46°	50°	59°	71°	78°	85°
Low	23°	25°	31°	39°	48°	56°
	JULY	AUG	SEPT	OCT	NOV	DEC
High	88°	86°	81°	71°	61°	50°
Low	60°	59°	52°	41°	34°	25°

Spring is the most variable season. During March, the first signs of rebirth appear in the lowlands, yet trees in the high country may not fully leaf out until June. Visitors can experience both winter- and summer-like weather in spring. As summer approaches, the strong fronts weaken, and thunderstorms and haze become more frequent. Summertime rainy days can be cool. In fall, continental fronts once again sweep through, clearing the air and bringing warm days and cool nights, though rain is always possible.

The first snows of winter usually arrive in November, and snow can intermittently fall through April, though no permanent snowpack exists. About 40 to 120 inches of snow can fall during this time. Expect to incur entire days of below-freezing weather, though temperatures can range from mild to bitterly cold.

Trail Selection

Four criteria were used during the selection of trails for this guide. Only the premier dayhikes and overnight backpacks are included, based upon most beautiful scenery, unique Shenandoah features, ease of access, and diversity of experience. Some of the selected trails are very popular; others are used infrequently. If you are fortunate enough to complete all the hikes in this book, you will gain a comprehensive appreciation for the complex beauty of an American gem of a national park.

Key Features

Top Trails books contain information about "features" for each trail, such as old-growth trees, waterfalls, great views, and more. Shenandoah National Park is blessed with an incredible diversity of terrain and associated flora and fauna—no matter what your interests, you're sure to find a trail to match them. Hikes range throughout the vast variety of ecosystems, from the spruce-fir pockets to the great oak forests to the deep canyons where verdant streams house waterfalls tumbling still deeper into the back of beyond. Those who love a view will find plenty of rock outcrops, meadows, and other vista points where rewarding views can be had. Photographers will be glad we live in the age of the digital camera, since they can shoot limitless pictures of showy spring wildflowers and vibrant fall color panoramas.

Campgrounds, cabins, and lodges throughout the park make for great base camps for hikers. Backcountry camping allows hikers to extend their trips beyond dayhiking. Anglers can toss a line in more than 50 fishable waterways. Plus some Shenandoah streams harbor swimming holes. Wildlife can be seen in the clearings of Big Meadows and other places between.

Multiple Uses

All the trails described in this guide are suitable for hiking. Some of the trails can also be enjoyed by equestrians, though the number of horseback enthusiasts in Shenandoah is far outstripped by hikers. Very few trails have more than sporadic equestrian use, though the Skyland area offers guided rides during the warm season. Bicyclists are relegated to Skyline Drive and paved roads, except for a mile-long stretch of Rapidan Fire Road. Fishing is done primarily along backcountry streams.

Unlike most national parks, *pets are allowed on the vast majority of backcountry trails,* but they must be on a six-foot leash. Certain paths that don't allow pets are signed as such and are noted in the trails table (page viii).

On the Trail

Every outing should begin with proper preparation, which usually takes only a few minutes. Even the easiest trail can turn up unexpected surprises. People seldom think about getting lost or injured, but unexpected things can and do happen. Simple precautions can make the difference between a good story and a dangerous situation.

Use the Top Trails ratings and descriptions to determine if a particular trail is a good match with your fitness and energy levels, given current conditions and the time of year.

Have a Plan

Choose Wisely The first step to enjoying any trail is to match the trail to your abilities. It's no use overestimating your experience or fitness—know your abilities and limitations, and use the Top Trails difficulty rating that accompanies each trail.

Leave Word about Your Plans The most basic of precautions is leaving word of your intentions with friends or family. Many people will hike the backcountry their entire lives without ever relying on this safety net, but establishing this simple habit is free insurance.

It's best to leave specific information—location, trail name, intended time of travel—with a responsible person. However, if this is not possible or if plans change at the last minute, you should still leave word. If there is a registration process available, make use of it. If there is a ranger station, trail register, or visitor center, check in.

Prepare and Plan

- Know your abilities and your limitations.
- Leave word about your plans with family and friends.
- Know the area and the route.

Review the Route Before embarking on any hike, read the entire description and study the map. It isn't necessary to memorize every detail, but it is worthwhile to have a clear mental picture of the trail and the general area. If the trail or terrain are complex, augment the trail guide with a topographic map. Maps and current weather and trail-condition information are often available from local ranger and park stations.

Carry the Essentials

Proper preparation for any type of trail use includes gathering certain essential items to carry. Your trip checklist will vary according to trail choice and conditions.

Trail Essentials

- Dress to keep cool, but be ready for cold.
- Bring plenty of water and adequate food.

Clothing When the weather is good, light, comfortable clothing is the obvious choice. It's easy to believe that very little spare clothing is needed, but a prepared hiker has something tucked away for any emergency from a surprise shower to an unexpected overnight in a remote area.

Clothing includes proper footwear, essential for hiking and running trails. As a trail becomes more demanding, you will need footwear that performs. Running shoes are fine for many trails. If you will be carrying substantial weight or encountering sustained rugged terrain, step up to hiking boots.

Shenandoah can be notoriously humid in summer. Hikers often sweat more than normal. Breathable, moisture-wicking clothes will help keep you cool and dry. In cooler weather, particularly when it's wet, carry waterproof outer garments and quick-drying undergarments (avoid cotton). Shenandoah can also be a rainy place. Unless the forecast calls for absolutely no chance of rain, bring a rain jacket or poncho. As general rule, whatever the conditions, bring layers that can be combined or removed to provide comfort and protection from the elements in a wide variety of conditions.

Water Never embark on a trail without carrying water. At all times, particularly in warm weather, adequate water is of key importance. Experts recommend at least two quarts of water per day, and when hiking in heat a gallon or more may be more appropriate. At the extreme, dehydration can be life threatening. More commonly, inadequate water brings fatigue and muscle aches.

For most outings, unless the day is very hot or the trail very long, you should plan to carry sufficient water for the entire trail. Unfortunately, in North America natural water sources are questionable, generally loaded with various risks: bacteria, viruses, and fertilizers.

Water Treatment If it's necessary to make use of trailside water, you should filter or treat it. There are three methods for treating water: boiling, chemical treatment, and filtering. Boiling is best, but often impractical—it requires a heat source, a pot, and time. Chemical treatments, available in sporting goods stores, handle some problems, including the troublesome *Giardia* parasite, but will not combat many artificial chemical pollutants. The preferred method is filtration, which removes *Giardia* and other contaminants and doesn't leave any unpleasant aftertaste.

If this hasn't convinced you to carry all the water you need, one final admonishment: Be prepared for surprises. Water sources described in the text or on maps can change course or dry up completely. Never run your water bottle dry in expectation of the next source; fill up when water is available and always keep a little in reserve.

Food While not as critical as water, food is energy and its importance shouldn't be underestimated. Avoid foods that are hard to digest, such as candy bars and potato chips. Carry high energy, fast-digesting foods: nutrition bars, dehydrated fruit, gorp, and jerky. Bring a little extra food—it's good protection against an outing that turns unexpectedly long, perhaps because of inclement weather or losing your way.

Useful But Less than Essential Items

Map and Compass (and the Know-How to Use Them) Many trails don't require much navigation, meaning a map and compass aren't always as essential as water or food—but it can be a close call. If the trail is remote or infrequently visited, a map and compass should be considered necessities.

A handheld GPS (Global Positioning System) receiver is also a useful trail companion, but is really no substitute for a map and compass. However, a GPS downloaded with topographic maps can be a real help. The hazard is batteries dying or the device otherwise becoming unusable. A map and compass don't require batteries.

Cell Phone Much of the Blue Ridge and lowlands near towns and along the roads that cross Shenandoah have some level of cellular coverage. However, in many areas, especially in hollows and along streams, there is no phone service. In extreme circumstances, a cell phone can be a lifesaver. But don't depend on it; coverage is too unpredictable and batteries fail. And be sure that the occasion warrants the phone call—a blister doesn't justify a call to search-and-rescue.

Gear Depending on the remoteness and rigor of the trail, there are many additional useful items to consider: pocketknife, flashlight, fire source (waterproof matches, light, or flint), and a first-aid kit. Every member of your party should carry the appropriate essential items described above; groups often split up or get separated along the trail. Solo hikers should be even more disciplined about preparation and carry more gear. Traveling solo is inherently more risky. This isn't meant to discourage solo travel, simply to emphasize the need for extra preparation.

Trail Etiquette

The overriding rule on the trail is "Leave No Trace." Interest in visiting natural areas continues to increase in North America, even as the quantity of unspoiled natural areas continues to shrink. These pressures make it ever more critical that we leave no trace of our visits.

Never Litter If you carried it in, it's easy enough to carry it out. Leave the trail in the same, if not better, condition in which you find it. Try picking up any litter you encounter and packing it out—it's a great feeling! Just one piece of garbage and you've made a difference.

Stay on the Trail Paths have been created, sometimes over many years, for many purposes: to protect the surrounding natural areas, to avoid dangers, and to provide the best route. Leaving the trail can cause damage that takes years to undo. Never cut switchbacks. Shortcutting rarely saves energy or time, and it takes a terrible toll on the land, trampling plant life and hastening erosion. Moreover, safety and consideration intersect on the trail. It's hard to get truly lost if you stay on the trail.

Share the Trail The best trails attract many visitors, and you should be prepared to share the trail with others. Do your part to minimize impact.

Trail Etiquette

- Leave no trace. Never litter.
- Stay on the trail. Never cut switchbacks.
- Share the trail. Use courtesy and commonsense.
- Leave it there. Don't disturb wildlife.

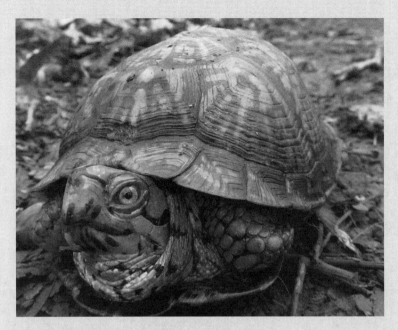

Even turtles *love the trails of Shenandoah.*

Commonly accepted trail etiquette dictates that **hikers yield to horseback riders, downhill hikers yield to uphill hikers, and everyone stays to the right.** Not everyone knows these rules of the road, so let commonsense and good humor be the final guide.

Leave It There Destruction or removal of plants and animals or historical, prehistoric, or geological items is certainly unethical and almost always illegal.

Getting Lost If you become lost on the trail, stay on the trail. Stop and take stock of the situation. In many cases, a few minutes of calm reflection will yield a solution. Consider all the clues available; use the sun to identify directions if you don't have a compass. If you determine that you are indeed lost, stay on the main trail and stay put. You are more likely to encounter other people if you stay in one place.

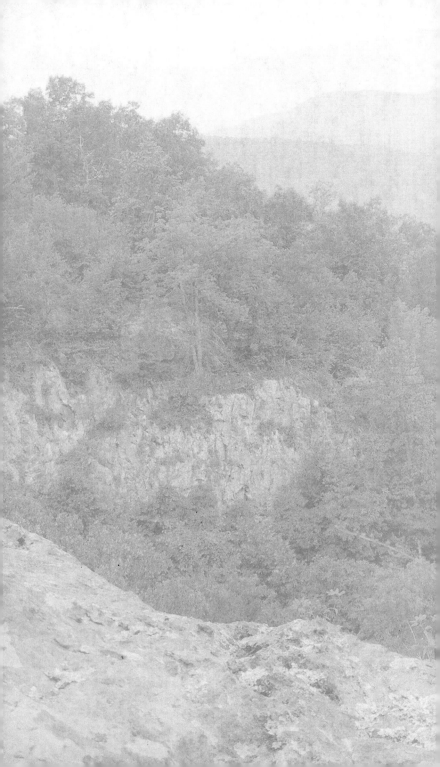

CHAPTER 1

North District

1. Dickey Ridge Historic Hike
2. Compton Peak
3. Big Devils Stairs Vista
4. Sugarloaf Loop
5. Overall Run Falls
6. Little Devils Stairs Loop
7. Traces Nature Trail
8. Overall Run Loop
9. Heiskell Hollow Loop
10. Elkwallow Loop
11. Piney River Falls
12. Knob Mountain and Jeremys Run Loop
13. Neighbor Mountain and Jeremys Run Loop
14. Thornton River Loop

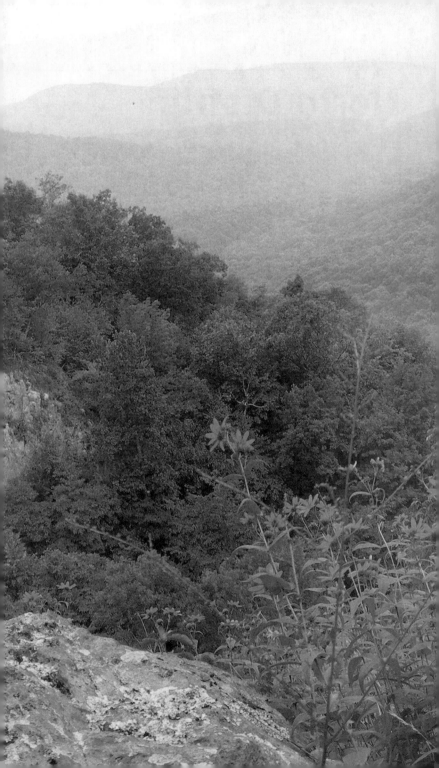

North District

The North District encompasses the most northerly of Shenandoah's three ranger districts that divide the park. This section stretches from Front Royal, the northernmost boundary of Shenandoah, to Thornton Gap in the south, where US 211 bisects the park while connecting Luray to Sperryville. Traveling south from Front Royal the Blue Ridge rises with proverbial Skyline Drive winding atop it. Dickey Ridge Visitor Center is often a hiker's first stop. A popular walk starts here. South of Dickey Ridge, notable heights, Compton Peak among others, begin rising where you can see the Blue Ridge rising from adjacent lowlands.

The park widens near Mount Marshall, and then you reach Mathews Arm Campground. Here, several streams and ridges spill off both sides of the Blue Ridge, creating a large wildland. On the west side of the Blue Ridge you find Overall Run Falls—the park's highest at 93 feet—tumbling over a ragged cliff. Remote Knob Mountain and Neighbor Mountain border ultrascenic Jeremys Run, with its big pools, waterfalls, swimming holes, and everywhere-you-look beauty. The Big Devils Stairs and Little Devils Stairs are boulder-covered, rugged gorges passable only by hikers. The Piney River cuts a secluded swath between Pignut Mountain and Piney Ridge, while the North Fork Thornton River Valley recalls pioneer history with its numerous homesites. Area streams have mostly trout, but some smallmouth bass. Sycamore, white pines, and mountain laurel, along with alder thickets, border the waterways. Shenandoah's famous oak stands rise on drier ridges. Elevations range from 550 feet near Front Royal to almost 3,400 feet atop Mount Marshall, in this, the smallest of the park's three districts.

The Appalachian Trail (AT) acts a spinal pathway for the North District, connecting all major watersheds, the mountains that divide them, and the trails that course through points high and low. The AT is useful for planning loop hikes in the North District. Most hikes here are accessed from Skyline Drive.

Overleaf and opposite: Vista from outcrop *near Overall Run Falls, on the Overall Run Trail (Trail 5)*

Visitors have one overnight option in the North District—Mathews Arm Campground. You can camp here on a first-come, first-served basis, but reservations are available on one loop. The higher elevation keeps it a good 10 degrees cooler than the Shenandoah Valley below. Make sure and store your food carefully, since Mathews Arm is bear country. More civilized accommodations can be had in nearby Front Royal or Luray.

The hikes described are either loops or out-and-back treks. Along the way you can see local highlights—Little Devils Stairs, Piney River Falls, and the old farms on Dickey Ridge. Other treks travel lesser trod trails, such as Sugarloaf and Beecher Ridge, where park beauty is more subtle.

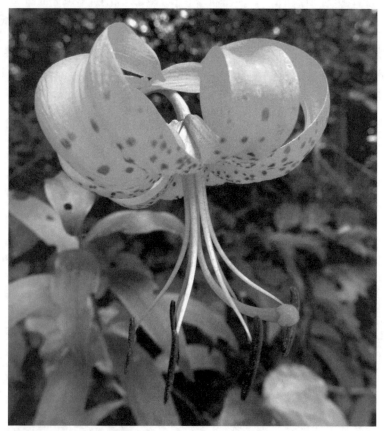

Turk's cap lily *graces the late summer forest on Big Devils Stairs Trail (Trail 3).*

Permits

Permits are not required for dayhiking. Backpackers must get a permit to stay in the backcountry. Simple self-registration stations are located at the Front Royal Entrance Station, Dickey Ridge Visitor Center, the north boundary where the AT leaves the park, and the Panorama and Thornton Gap Entrance Station.

Maps

For the North District, here are the USGS 7.5-minute (1:24,000-scale) topographic quadrangles that you will need, listed in the order that you will need them as you hike along your route.

Trail 1: *Chester Gap* and *Front Royal*
Trail 2: *Chester Gap*
Trail 3: *Chester Gap*
Trail 4: *Bentonville* and *Thornton Gap*
Trail 5: *Bentonville*
Trail 6: *Thornton Gap* and *Bentonville*
Trail 7: *Bentonville*
Trail 8: *Bentonville*
Trail 9: *Bentonville*
Trail 10: *Bentonville* and *Thornton Gap*
Trail 11: *Thornton Gap*
Trail 12: *Thornton Gap* and *Bentonville*
Trail 13: *Thornton Gap*
Trail 14: *Thornton Gap*

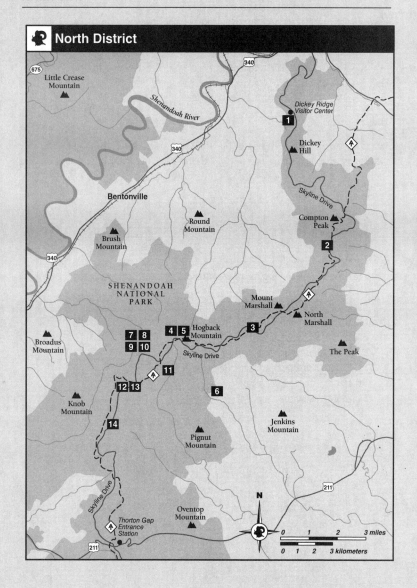

North District

TRAIL FEATURES TABLE

North District

TRAIL	Difficulty	Length	Type	USES & ACCESS	TERRAIN	NATURE	OTHER
1	2	4.3	Loop	Dayhiking, Pets Prohibited	Ridgeline	Autumn Colors	Great Views, Historic Interest
2	3	3.2	Out & Back	Dayhiking	Summit, Ridgeline	Autumn Colors	Great Views, Geologic Interest
3	3	5.0	Out & Back	Dayhiking, Backpacking	Ridgeline, Stream	Autumn Colors, Wildflowers	Great Views
4	3	4.7	Loop	Dayhiking, Backpacking	Ridgeline, Stream	Autumn Colors, Wildflowers, Wildlife	Great Views, Geologic Interest
5	4	6.8	Out & Back	Dayhiking	Ridgeline, Stream, Waterfall	Autumn Colors, Wildflowers, Wildlife	Great Views, Geologic Interest
6	4	5.4	Loop	Dayhiking, Backpacking	Ridgeline, Stream, Waterfall	Autumn Colors, Wildflowers	Great Views, Geologic Interest, Historic Interest
7	2	1.6	Loop	Dayhiking, Child-Friendly	Ridgeline	Autumn Colors	Historic Interest
8	5	9.2	Loop	Backpacking, Backpacking	Ridgeline, Stream, Waterfall	Autumn Colors, Wildlife	Great Views, Geologic Interest, Historic Interest, Swimming, Secluded, Steep
9	4	7.2	Loop	Dayhiking, Backpacking	Ridgeline, Stream	Autumn Colors, Wildflowers, Wildlife	Historic Interest, Secluded
10	3	5.6	Loop	Dayhiking	Ridgeline, Stream	Autumn Colors, Wildflowers, Wildlife	Secluded
11	4	6.8	Out & Back	Dayhiking, Backpacking	Ridgeline, Stream, Waterfall	Autumn Colors	Secluded
12	5	13.1	Loop	Dayhiking, Backpacking	Summit, Ridgeline, Stream, Waterfall	Autumn Colors, Wildlife	Great Views, Geologic Interest, Swimming, Steep
13	5	14.0	Loop	Dayhiking, Backpacking	Summit, Ridgeline, Stream, Waterfall	Autumn Colors, Wildflowers	Great Views, Swimming, Secluded, Steep
14	4	7.9	Loop	Dayhiking, Backpacking	Summit, Ridgeline, Stream	Autumn Colors, Wildflowers, Wildlife	Historic Interest, Secluded

Legend

USES & ACCESS
- Dayhiking
- Backpacking
- Child-Friendly
- Pets Prohibited

TYPE
- Loop
- Out & Back
- DIFFICULTY - 1 2 3 4 5 + (less ... more)

TERRAIN
- Summit
- Ridgeline
- Stream
- Waterfall

NATURE
- Autumn Colors
- Wildflowers
- Wildlife
- Old-Growth

FEATURES
- Great Views
- Geologic Interest
- Historic Interest
- Swimming
- Secluded
- Steep

North District

TRAIL 1

Dayhiking,
Pets Prohibited
4.3 miles, Loop
Difficulty: 1 **2** 3 4 5

Dickey Ridge Historic Hike 27
Easy access, old farmsteads, and a good view sum
up much of what Shenandoah National Park offers
in one hike. Leave Dickey Ridge Visitor Center, and
slip down to the old Fox Farm. Discover pioneer
vestiges there, including a cemetery. Walk south
on Dickey Ridge to Snead Farm site, and check
out more human history. Catch a great view of the
Shenandoah Valley on your way back, then enjoy
more attractive ridgeline woodland.

TRAIL 2

Dayhiking
3.2 miles, Out & Back
Difficulty: 1 2 **3** 4 5

Compton Peak 33
This hike takes a lesser-used approach to a mountaintop with two rewarding vistas from rock protrusions
along its flanks. The Appalachian Trail climbs moderately to these panoramas. Along the way explore
nature's recovery and fire ecology, where the Smith
Run Fire enveloped 1,710 acres of the park.

TRAIL 3

Dayhiking, Backpacking
5.0 miles, Out & Back
Difficulty: 1 2 **3** 4 5

Big Devils Stairs Vista 37
This moderate hike leads to a great reward, with
plenty of solitude along the way. The nearly level
Bluff Trail leads to the Big Devils Stairs canyon rim
for a deep view of the valley below and the mountains beyond. At the hike's outset, pass a shelter used
by long-distance hikers on the Appalachian Trail.

Sugarloaf Loop 43

Drop off the eastern side of Hogback Mountain into the upper Piney River Valley. Relish far-reaching views on the Appalachian Trail, then follow a moderate grade into the Piney River on the Sugarloaf Trail. A grassy flat beside the Piney River makes for a great resting spot. Return to the high country, soaking in more great views from Hogback Mountain before closing the loop.

TRAIL 4

Dayhiking, Backpacking
4.7 miles, Loop
Difficulty: 1 2 **3** 4 5

Overall Run Falls 49

Hike to the park's highest falls and a grand vista beyond. Start with a mountaintop stroll on the Appalachian Trail, wending down the slopes of Hogback Mountain, crossing many flats. Find Twin Falls, then come to Overall Run Falls. From a rocky precipice, you can see the nearby cataract and the Appalachian splendor in the distance.

TRAIL 5

Dayhiking
6.8 miles, Out & Back
Difficulty: 1 2 3 **4** 5

Little Devils Stairs Loop 55

This rewarding hike delivers every step you take. You undertake the challenging part—ascending Little Devils Stairs Canyon—at the beginning. Absorb beauty everywhere you look in this rough canyon. After emerging from the upper canyon, take Keyser Run Fire Road to enjoy a highland vista, then view pioneer internment Bolen Cemetery along the way.

TRAIL 6

Dayhiking, Backpacking
5.4 miles, Loop
Difficulty: 1 2 3 **4** 5

Traces Nature Trail 61

Where yesteryear's Virginians made a life, you can now follow a recreational path wandering through high-country woods. This hike encircling Mathews Arm Campground reveals traces of pioneer settlements dating back to before this national park came to be.

TRAIL 7

Dayhiking,
Child-Friendly,
Pets Prohibited
1.6 miles, Loop
Difficulty: 1 **2** 3 4 5

TRAIL 8

Dayhiking, Backpacking
9.2 miles, Loop
Difficulty: 1 2 3 4 **5**

Overall Run Loop 67

This challenging loop drops more than 2,000 feet, and then climbs back up, every foot. Join remote Beecher Ridge, making a glorious walk through lush forests before dropping to Overall Run. Work upstream in a rugged gorge, passing a superlative swimming hole. Come to Overall Run Falls, the park's highest at 93 feet. Observe this cataract, and enjoy a mountain panorama before finishing the circuit.

TRAIL 9

Dayhiking, Backpacking
7.2 miles, Loop
Difficulty: 1 2 3 **4** 5

Heiskell Hollow Loop 73

This Mathews Arm area trek has no single superlative feature to draw in hikers but offers solitude aplenty. Hike secluded Beecher Ridge, traveling the spine of this regally forested highland before picking up the Heiskell Hollow Trail. Plenty of pioneer evidence awaits a sharp-eyed hiker.

TRAIL 10

Dayhiking
5.6 miles, Loop
Difficulty: 1 2 **3** 4 5

Elkwallow Loop 77

This classic Shenandoah circuit first navigates a boulder field before making a pleasantly level highland track on the Blue Ridge. Eventually dip to Jeremys Run. Pick up the seldom-trod Knob Mountain Trail on a remarkably level track to finish the circuit.

TRAIL 11

Dayhiking, Backpacking
6.8 miles, Out & Back
Difficulty: 1 2 3 **4** 5

Piney River Falls 83

The scenery on this solitude-laden hike meets high Shenandoah standards, and the falls are a worthy destination. Gently wind your way through eye-pleasing, high-country woods to the Piney River Valley and the three-tier falls.

Knob Mountain and
Jeremys Run Loop 89

This is a long yet rewarding loop exploring points high and low. Traverse Knob Mountain, soaking in views en route to Jeremys Run. Make your way up gorgeous Jeremys Run valley, crossing the stream more than a dozen times. Don't expect company on Knob Mountain, though you may see a few people along Jeremys Run.

TRAIL 12

Dayhiking, Backpacking
13.1 miles, Loop
Difficulty: 1 2 3 4 **5**

Neighbor Mountain and
Jeremys Run Loop 95

This circuit leaves Elkwallow Picnic Area, southbound on the Appalachian Trail, traversing a pleasant stretch of the world's most famous pathway. Join secluded Neighbor Mountain Trail, and grab some views on your way to Jeremys Run, one of the prettiest and most productive trout streams in the park. Crisscross to the upper valley of Jeremys Run, then make a final climb, returning to the trailhead.

TRAIL 13

Dayhiking, Backpacking
14.0 miles, Loop
Difficulty: 1 2 3 4 **5**

Thornton River Loop 101

Make a quiet, solitude-rich hike through history, combined with high-country trekking. Enter once settled Thornton Hollow. Walk along alluring North Fork Thornton River, wandering richly forested flats between creek crossings. Leave the lowlands on the Hull School Trail, crossing Skyline Drive. Trace the Appalachian Trail on a pleasant track back to the trailhead.

TRAIL 14

Dayhiking, Backpacking
7.9 miles, Loop
Difficulty: 1 2 3 **4** 5

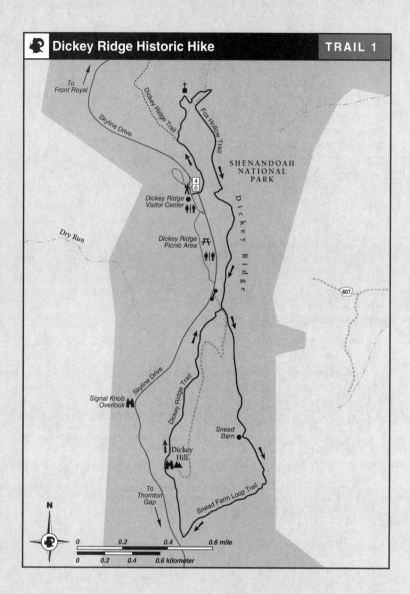

To Front Royal

Dickey Ridge Trail

Skyline Drive

Fox Hollow Trail

SHENANDOAH NATIONAL PARK

4/6

Dickey Ridge Visitor Center

Dickey Ridge

Dry Run

Dickey Ridge Picnic Area

607

Skyline Drive

Dickey Ridge Trail

Signal Knob Overlook

Snead Barn

Dickey Hill

To Thornton Gap

Snead Farm Loop Trail

N

0   0.2   0.4   0.6 mile

0   0.2   0.4   0.6 kilometer

Dickey Ridge Historic Hike

Easy access, old farmsteads, and a good view piece together a nice family or group hike that sums up much of what Shenandoah National Park offers. Leave the Dickey Ridge Visitor Center, and slip down to the old Fox Farm, which has many pioneer vestiges, including a cemetery. Walk south on Dickey Ridge. Walk south to the Snead Farm site, and check out more human history. Make a rewarding woodland walk. Catch a great view of the Shenandoah Valley on your way back, then enjoy more attractive hilltop woodland. *Note:* Pets are *not* allowed on this trail.

Best Time

After the leaves fall—winter through early spring—is the best time for this hike. This is when you can best see the ample evidence of pre-park residents. Summer can be warm and busy.

Finding the Trail

The hike starts at the Dickey Ridge Visitor Center, milepost 4.6 on Skyline Drive. From the Front Royal Entrance Station, head south on Skyline Drive for 4.6 miles to the visitor center.

Trail Description

Leave the visitor center near the flagpole. ▶1 Interestingly, the visitor center was originally a dining hall for a set of now-demolished rental cabins, built in the early days of Shenandoah National Park. Cross

TRAIL USE
Dayhiking,
Pets Prohibited

LENGTH
4.3 miles, 2½–3½ hours

CUMULATIVE
ELEVATION +/-
-700'/+700'

DIFFICULTY
– 1 **2** 3 4 5 +

TRAIL TYPE
Loop

START & FINISH
N38° 52.296'
W78° 12.273'

FEATURES
Ridgeline
Autumn Colors
Historic Interest
Great Views

FACILITIES
Visitor center
Restrooms
Water
Picnic tables

Skyline Drive. Easterly views open beyond the grassy hill in front of you. You can purchase an interpretive pamphlet here. Turn left at an informational sign, walk a short distance, then join the Dickey Ridge Trail, entering woodland. The hardwood forest here is covered in vines. At 0.3 mile, turn right on the Fox Hollow Nature Trail. ▶2 As you descend into Fox Hollow, you see walls of rock, relics of the farms that were here before the brushy woods that now occupy the site. Look at the large stone edifice, placed there by generations of Foxes toiling the terrain, clearing the land to increase fertility and yield. More rock walls stand down the trail.

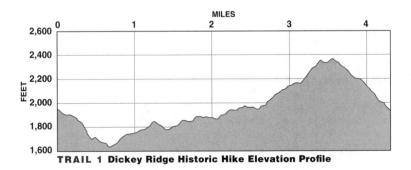 **Historic Interest**

At 0.5 mile, come to the Fox family cemetery. ▶3 Bordered by fieldstones and cloaked in periwinkle, the graveyard is a somber reminder that this land was many things to many people before it became a national park. The name Dickey Ridge appears in records dating back to before the United States was established. Soon pass a spring enclosed in concrete. This spring, once used by Foxes, was encased in concrete only after the national park drew water for the dining hall turned visitor center. Ahead, embedded in the ground, lies a decorative millstone, once made to grind corn elsewhere, but used as a decorative step by the Foxes. The trail

TRAIL 1 Dickey Ridge Historic Hike Elevation Profile

For a short historic stroll, walk the Dickey Ridge and Fox Hollow Loop, returning to the Dickey Ridge Visitor Center after 1.3 miles, with an elevation change of only 250 feet.

bisects the spring outflow and then switches back, passing a rusty wire fence.

It then picks up an old road connecting Dickey Ridge to Front Royal at 0.7 mile. The loop turns south and scrambles uphill in brushy woods before rejoining the Dickey Ridge Trail at 1.3 miles. ▶4 The visitor center stands just above you.

To continue the longer double loop, stay with the gentle Dickey Ridge Trail. It cruises through more vine-covered woods. Watch for a rock fence that runs along a steep slope left of the trail. There weren't many out-of-shape farmers in these Potomac Highlands. At 1.9 miles, reach the junction with Snead Farm Road. Turn left here, joining a blue-blazed gravel track. ▶5 Then come to three signed road forks. At the first fork, take the road to the left—the road right leads to a Federal Aviation Administration (FAA) flight-tracking station. At the second fork, take the road to the right—the left fork goes to the water station for Dickey Ridge Visitor Center and its picnic area. Just ahead, look for an old bricked-in spring to the right of the roadbed. At the third fork, take the road to the left. Stay under a transmission line.

At 2.4 miles, come to a clearing with the white Snead Barn and the concrete and stone foundation of a house. ▶6 Ol' Snead was a relative newcomer to what became the park. The former judge owned the place only a few years before the park bought him out. The function of the cellar behind the barn has been lost to time. Explore to find the spring.

At the edge of the clearing, turn left on the Snead Farm Loop Trail. This path runs level a short

▲ **Ridgeline**

Explore Shenandoah's past on this great family hike.

Autumn Colors

Great Views

distance, then makes an irregular climb in rocky hardwoods before meeting the Dickey Ridge Trail at 3.2 miles. ▶7 Turn right on the Dickey Ridge Trail, topping out in 0.3 mile. Stay left here as a trail leads right to the top of a knob and the FAA airplane tracking station. Leave it be. The trail descends. At 3.6 miles, come to a cleared overlook of the Shenandoah Valley, South Fork Shenandoah River, and Massanutten Mountain. ▶8

The trail rises briefly once again before making a prolonged descent through a very pleasant forest of oak, hickory, maple, basswood, and other trees. Reach Snead Farm Road and the Dickey Ridge Trail at 4.3 miles. ▶9 From here, it is about a half-mile meander back through the grass and trees of the Dickey Ridge Picnic Area. This mileage is not included in the overall hike, since there are multiple routes through the picnic ground.

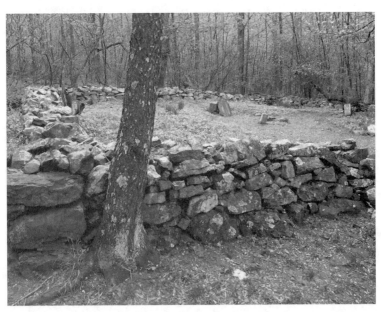

Primitive stone walls *border the cemetery at Fox Farm.*

🚶 MILESTONES

▶1	0.0	Dickey Ridge Visitor Center at milepost 4.6
▶2	0.3	Right on Fox Hollow Trail
▶3	0.5	Fox Cemetery
▶4	1.3	Complete Fox Hollow Loop, and go straight on Dickey Ridge Trail
▶5	1.9	Left on Snead Farm Road
▶6	2.4	Snead Barn and homesite
▶7	3.2	Right on Dickey Ridge Trail
▶8	3.6	Vista
▶9	4.3	Reach Snead Farm Road and Dickey Ridge Trail at south end of picnic area. Meander back to visitor center.

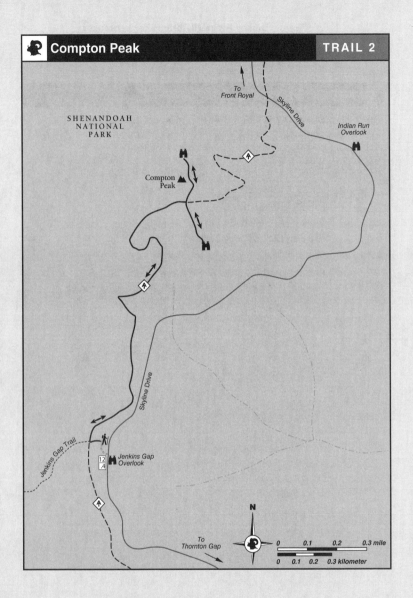

SHENANDOAH
NATIONAL
PARK

To
Front Royal

Skyline Drive

Indian Run
Overlook

Compton
Peak

Skyline Drive

Jenkins Gap Trail

12
4

Jenkins Gap
Overlook

To
Thornton Gap

N

0　　　0.1　　　0.2　　　0.3 mile

0　　0.1　　0.2　　0.3 kilometer

Compton Peak

This out-and-back dayhike takes the lesser-used approach to a mountaintop with two good vistas from rock protrusions along its flanks. The Appalachian Trail (AT) is your host along the way to these two outcrops. Additionally, you can explore fire ecology, since this shaping force of Shenandoah National Park swept over Compton Peak in February 2011. The Smith Run Fire eventually enveloped 1,710 acres of the park, primarily west of Skyline Drive in the Jenkins Gap area, where this hike starts. A landowner adjacent to the park improperly dumped ashes from his woodstove, and the fire ensued.

Best Time

For this highland vista hike, the clearer the sky, the better the views.

Finding the Trail

From Front Royal, take Skyline Drive south for 12.4 miles to the Jenkins Gap parking area, located on the right at milepost 12.4 on Skyline Drive, just before the Jenkins Gap Overlook, which is on the left (east). The hike starts on the Jenkins Gap Trail, which leaves from the parking area, not the overlook.

Trail Description

Begin this walk on the Jenkins Gap Trail. ▶1 The yellow-blazed pathway leaves from the parking area around auto-sized boulders to intersect the

TRAIL USE
Dayhiking
LENGTH
3.2 miles, 2–3 hours
CUMULATIVE ELEVATION +/-
+560'/-560'
DIFFICULTY
– 1 2 **3** 4 5 +
TRAIL TYPE
Out & Back
START & FINISH
N38° 48.395'
W78° 10.854'

FEATURES
Great Views
Autumn Colors
Ridgeline
Summit
Geologic Interest

FACILITIES
None

33

AT in 164 feet. Turn right, heading northbound. The walking is easy in a mixed forest of sassafras, pin cherry, locust, and ever-present oak, shading a brushy forest floor. Look for partially blackened trunks of trees and other burn evidence. Of course, the woods are growing back well, albeit thick and brushy. Plenty of tall trees survived the burn. Keep a level track through Jenkins Gap. Skyline Drive lies to your right. After a while you may begin to wonder about the climb to Compton Peak. Finally, after 0.5 mile, the trail veers left and ascends a mountainside of chestnut oak and mountain laurel. ▶2

🌺 **Autumn Colors**

🔺 **Ridgeline**

Swing around the southwest side of Compton Peak. Switchback on some elaborate stone steps built during a trail reroute. The trail regains the ridgecrest. Southward views of North Mount Marshall and South Mount Marshall open. Step over a little spring branch at 0.9 mile. ▶3 Look for apple trees persisting in the forest beyond the spring. These are remnants of an orchard on the north and south side of Jenkins Gap. I have seen a bear harvesting apples while hiking here during late summer. The AT curves past the head of the spring, angling higher.

🧍 **Summit**

Pass through a flat then climb a bit more to reach a four-way trail junction at 1.3 miles. ▶4 Both left and right lead to vistas. Head left on the blue-blazed

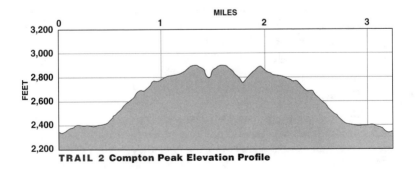

TRAIL 2 Compton Peak Elevation Profile

trail, to the more popular and widespread view. Briefly continue climbing a stony track over a rock knob before dipping to an outcrop with a widespread vista at 1.5 miles. ►5 Below, the track of Skyline Drive, including Gooney Run Overlook, is evident as it snakes downhill along Dickey Ridge. To the far left are the South Fork of the Shenandoah River and the Shenandoah Valley. Ahead, more mountains and the flatlands extend toward Washington, D.C. This is a truly inspiring vista.

The second vista is more challenging to reach and less inspiring. If you have made it this far, go ahead and check out the second view. Backtrack to reach the AT and keep forward, now on the second blue-blazed path. The trail is fainter as it goes down, down, down on a rocky tread. Reach an outcrop where you might expect a vista, but keep hiking. Hike down the bluff, walk a few feet through the woods, and scramble up a rocky prominence at mile 1.9. ►6 This prominence, an example of columnar jointing, offers worthy views of Mount Marshall in the foreground and lands east of the Blue Ridge. While thinking of the unfortunate people who skip this second view, as evidenced by its less-used trail, the return trip to the AT will get you huffing and puffing. The blue-blazed trail now leads to the base of this prominence and then dead-ends. ►7

 Great Views

 Great Views

> This climb to a first-rate vista isn't too steep.

🚶	**MILESTONES**	
►1	0.0	Jenkins Gap Trail parking area at milepost 12.4
►2	0.5	Ascend from Jenkins Gap
►3	0.9	Spring
►4	1.3	Four-way split to vistas
►5	1.5	Northwest vista
►6	1.9	Southeast vista
►7	3.2	Jenkins Gap Trail parking area at milepost 12.4

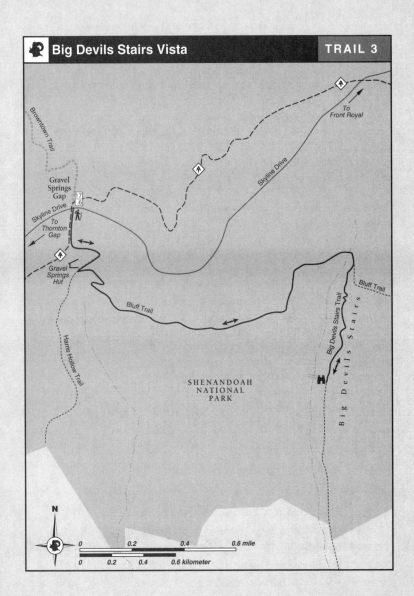

Big Devils Stairs Vista

TRAIL 3

Browntown Trail

To Front Royal

Skyline Drive

Gravel
Springs
Gap

17
6

Skyline Drive

To
Thornton
Gap

Gravel
Springs
Hut

Bluff Trail

Bluff Trail

Big Devils Stairs Trail

Big Devils Stairs

Harris Hollow Trail

SHENANDOAH
NATIONAL
PARK

N

| 0 | 0.2 | 0.4 | 0.6 mile |

| 0 | 0.2 | 0.4 | 0.6 kilometer |

Big Devils Stairs Vista

This is a moderate hike with a great reward. The walking is easy, and the trails are used surprisingly little. The nearly level Bluff Trail leads to the Big Devils Stairs canyon rim for a great view of the valley below and the mountains beyond. At the hike's outset, you will pass a shelter used by long-distance hikers on the Appalachian Trail (AT).

Best Time

Even though this hike culminates in a view, it is primarily of a canyon, rather than distant mountains and valleys. Therefore, it is good any time of year.

Finding the Trail

The Gravel Springs Gap parking area is at milepost 17.6 on the east side of Skyline Drive. The yellow-blazed access road to Gravel Springs Hut leaves the rear of the parking area.

Trail Description

A large trailhead signboard shows the web of paths in the immediate area. Leave Skyline Drive from the rear of the Gravel Springs Gap parking area on the gated access road leading down to Gravel Springs Hut. ►1 The AT leaves from the parking area as well. The southbound portion of the AT roughly parallels the access road, while the northbound AT crosses Skyline Drive here at Gravel Springs Gap. The walking is easy on the fire road, bordered

TRAIL USE
Dayhiking, Backpacking

LENGTH
5.0 miles, 3–4 hours

CUMULATIVE
ELEVATION +/-
-690'/+690'

DIFFICULTY
− 1 2 **3** 4 5 +

TRAIL TYPE
Out & Back

START & FINISH
N38° 46.085'
W78° 14.000'

FEATURES
Stream
Ridgeline
Wildflowers
Autumn Colors
Great Views

FACILITIES
None

by locust, apple trees, and ample brush. You are working downhill.

After a quarter mile, the trail makes a switchback to the left and the Harris Hollow Trail leads left to the Bluff Trail, your destination. The horse trail allows equestrian access to the Bluff Trail without going to Gravel Springs Hut. Stay right with the roadbed, drifting down to Gravel Springs at 0.4 mile. ►2 You will see the rocked-in upwelling to your right. The three-sided trail shelter, fronted by a fireplace, stands just beyond. Primarily of stone and wood construction, these trail shelters are based roughly 10 miles apart the entire length of the AT, including here at Shenandoah National Park. Imagine staying in shelters like this one on the 2,100-mile trek from Georgia to Maine.

This hike continues on the Bluff Trail, which leaves the shelter clearing near Gravel Springs. Pass the Harris Hollow Trail coming from Gravel Springs Gap. Make a big switchback ahead, stepping over a spring branch. At 0.6 mile, the Harris Hollow Trail leaves right. Again, the Harris Hollow Trail is confusingly working around Gravel Springs and the trail shelter so that horses won't foul the spring. Stay with the Bluff Trail, recrossing the spring branch. From here, it runs nearly level,

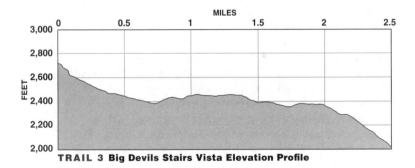

TRAIL 3 Big Devils Stairs Vista Elevation Profile

around 2,300 feet, on the southeast slope of Mount Marshall beneath a high-canopied forest of multitrunked basswood, oak, and hickory strewn with large boulders, low bluffs, and outcrops.

 Wildflowers

At 1.1 miles, the forest opens on the right amid rock, offering views to the south. Ahead, several branches cross the trail and meet the main stem flowing from Gravel Springs. They all ultimately flow into the Rush River, outside the park. Many of these will be dry in late summer and fall. At 1.8

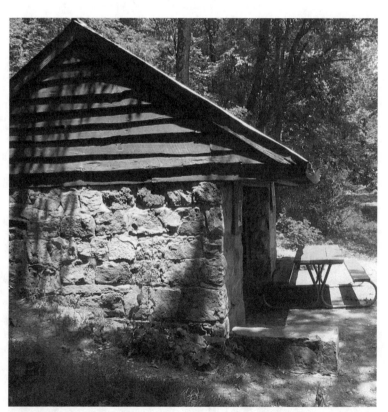

Gravel Springs Hut *is but one of many trail shelters scattered along the Appalachian Trail in Shenandoah and beyond.*

miles, step over the upper reaches of the stream that runs through Big Devils Stairs Gorge, which is just beginning to cut its way down the mountainside. ►3 This unnamed tributary, also a branch of the Rush River, is an easy crossing in times of normal water flow. Enter a flat, then come to the Big Devils Stairs Trail junction at 1.9 miles. ►4

Stream

Turn right onto the Big Devils Stairs Trail, which follows the east rim of the gorge. Notice how abruptly the forest changes. The trees here are those typically found on drier south- or west-facing slopes—chestnut oak and Virginia pine—with an understory of mountain laurel. A scattering of pale white rock adds to the green mosaic. At 2.0 miles, the declining path makes a few switchbacks while meandering down the rim of the gorge.

Autumn Colors

Ridgeline

Your descent may leave you antsy about finding the outcrop with the view, especially when boulders to the right of the trail through the woods seem to offer vantages. Stay with the trail and you won't miss *the* view. After an abrupt right turn, the trail comes to the edge of the gorge. Continue down the trail on stone steps, and descend to a large rock outcrop at 2.5 miles. ►5 Grand views open of the Big Devils Stairs canyon and the mountains beyond. Look at the stone walls rising from the stream below! Listen to the stream crashing through boulders at the canyon bottom. Follow the trail along the rim of the gorge for more vistas.

Great Views

Ahead, another outcrop hosts a gnarled pine hanging from its edge. Enjoy more views of the beautiful Shenandoah country, including Pignut Mountain, Piney Ridge, and fields beyond the park bounds. After this vista, the trail begins a steep descent and is not recommended. There is no public access from the lower end of the Big Devils Stairs. A trail once ran straight up the canyon, but after repeatedly washing out it was rerouted on the rim where you stand.

🚶	**MILESTONES**		
▶1	0.0	Gravel Springs Gap parking area at milepost 17.6
▶2	0.4	Gravel Springs Hut
▶3	1.8	Cross stream of Big Devils Stairs canyon
▶4	1.9	Right on Big Devils Stairs Trail
▶5	2.5	Big Devils Stairs vista

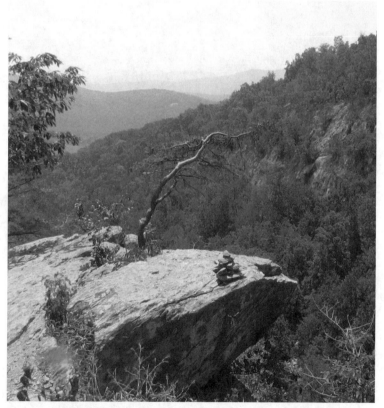

Big Devils Stairs Canyon *cuts a chasm while ridges rise beyond.*

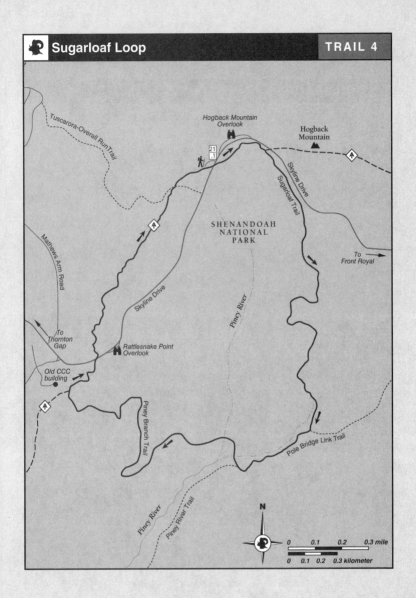

Tuscarora-Overall Run Trail

Hogback Mountain
Overlook

Hogback
Mountain

21
.1

SHENANDOAH
NATIONAL
PARK

Skyline Drive

Sugarloaf Trail

Mathews Arm Road

Skyline Drive

To
Front Royal

To
Thornton
Gap

Piney River

Rattlesnake Point
Overlook

Old CCC
building

Piney Branch Trail

Pole Bridge Link Trail

Piney River

Piney River Trail

N

| 0 | 0.1 | 0.2 | 0.3 mile |

| 0 | 0.1 | 0.2 | 0.3 kilometer |

Sugarloaf Loop

This loop dips off the eastern side of Hogback Mountain into the upper Piney River Valley. You will relish far-reaching views on the Appalachian Trail (AT), then follow a moderate grade into the Piney River on the Sugarloaf Trail. A grassy flat beside the Piney River makes for a great resting spot. Head back to the high country, soaking in more great views from Hogback Mountain before completing the loop.

Best Time

Spring through fall are the most rewarding. Wildflowers bloom in the valley during spring. Summer offers a cool and shady respite. Enjoy views on clear fall days, and you might spot wildlife on the trail.

Finding the Trail

The hike starts at the parking area just south of the Hogback Mountain Overlook, milepost 21.1 on Skyline Drive. To reach the trailhead from the Thornton Gap Entrance Station, take Skyline Drive north for 10.4 miles to the parking area on the west side of Skyline Drive, just before Hogback Mountain Overlook. The loop hike starts on the eastern side of Skyline Drive where the AT crosses Skyline Drive.

Trail Description

From the parking area just south of Hogback Overlook, pick up the AT, northbound, as it crosses

TRAIL USE
Dayhiking, Backpacking

LENGTH
4.7 miles, 3–4 hours

**CUMULATIVE
ELEVATION +/-**
-870'/+870'

DIFFICULTY
– 1 2 **3** 4 5 +

TRAIL TYPE
Loop

START & FINISH
N38° 45.627'
W78° 16.953'

FEATURES
Stream
Ridgeline
Autumn Colors
Geologic Interest
Wildlife
Great Views

FACILITIES
None

over to the eastern side of Skyline Drive. ▶1 Hike through fern-floored oak woods, shortly climbing to a rocky knob spiked with uptilted rock. Note the rock combination to the right of the trail that resembles a chair. Many a hiker has had their picture taken in that oversized throne. At 0.2 mile, a side trail leads left to a rock outcrop framed in mountain ash trees. ▶2 The western vistas are extensive. Hogback Mountain Overlook is immediately below you. Overall Run cuts a chasm. Ridges rise around it. The Shenandoah Valley stretches out past the park. Beyond the valley other mountains rise to frame the patchwork of farm, field, and town.

Geologic Interest

Great Views

Descend among rocky woods. Notice how the winds have sculpted the trees to face easterly. Reach the slender Sugarloaf Trail at 0.3 mile. ▶3 Here, turn right onto a single-track path lined with mountain laurel beneath scattered oaks. Briefly run parallel to Skyline Drive, joining an old wagon road. The Sugarloaf Trail curves back to the right, winding on a slightly sloped ridge, former pastureland. Descend to step over two rocky streamlets, wide but shallow feeder branches of the Piney River. Straight rock pioneer walls contrast with the fluid shapes of nature. Backpackers can find legal campsites off the trail in the next mile or so. This loop is a great

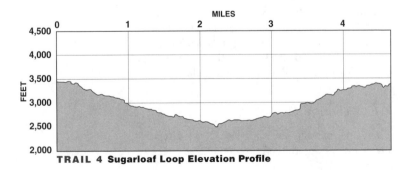

TRAIL 4 Sugarloaf Loop Elevation Profile

break-in trip for the novice overnighter and a quick, quality one-night getaway for everyone.

Reach a trail junction at mile 1.7. Turn right onto the Pole Bridge Link Trail. The land is level in these parts—for mountain land. It was cultivated too, despite the rocks you see. Pass through a changing forest, where hardwoods, such as black birch and yellow birch, are vying to replace the fallen hemlocks that once colored the vale evergreen. The gradual descent leads to another trail junction at 2.1 miles. Stay right with the Piney Branch Trail. ▶4

Step over the rocky branches you crossed earlier before reaching the upper Piney River in 0.1 mile. Large boulders and rocks line the watercourse. Cross the river to reach a grassy flat flanked by a large boulder. This locale makes a nice respite. A set of cascades downstream of this crossing are worth a look.

Leave this low point of the loop—you are now a little higher than 2,500 feet—and start climbing toward the crest of the Blue Ridge on a gentle grade. Big rocks line the trailbed. At mile 3.2, pass through an open area with a tremendous rock face rising up the hill to your right. ▶5 In September, bears converge and eat cherries from trees that grow nearby. You will see much purple, seed-laden bear scat along this path in the fall.

Curve uphill away from the roadbed to cross a second roadbed near a national park survey marker. The AT is just uphill, at 3.5 miles. Turn right onto the AT, making northbound tracks through open woodland where large widespread oaks grow over grass. ▶6 Younger trees view for sunlight. Undulate over a rocky hill to reach Skyline Drive at 3.7 miles. ▶7 Rattlesnake Point Overlook is just up road. Keep northbound, crossing Skyline Drive, and ascend the south side of Hogback Mountain.

A side trail at mile 4.0 leads left to an outcrop with views. ▶8 The ridgeline that is Massanutten

Stream

Geologic Interest

Wildlife

Ridgeline

Mountain forms a backdrop to South Fork Shenandoah River Valley. Range upon range of Shenandoah's mountains roll south. Dip into a pretty, grassy gap, then resume climbing to reach the Tuscarora-Overall Run Trail at mile 4.5. ►9 Pass a limited vista point on trail right before drifting into the parking area at mile 4.7, completing your loop. ►10

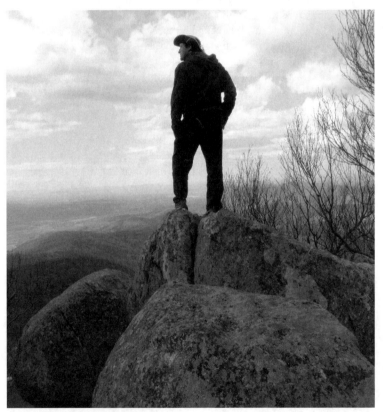

Surveying the mountain lands *west from a trailside overlook on the Appalachian Trail.*

🚶 MILESTONES

►1	0.0	Parking area at milepost 21.1
►2	0.2	View from Hogback Mountain
►3	0.3	Right on Sugarloaf Trail
►4	2.1	Stay right to join the Piney Branch Trail
►5	3.2	Pass rock face
►6	3.5	Right on the AT
►7	3.7	Cross Skyline Drive
►8	4.0	Vista
►9	4.5	Tuscarora-Overall Run Trail leaves left
►10	4.7	Complete loop

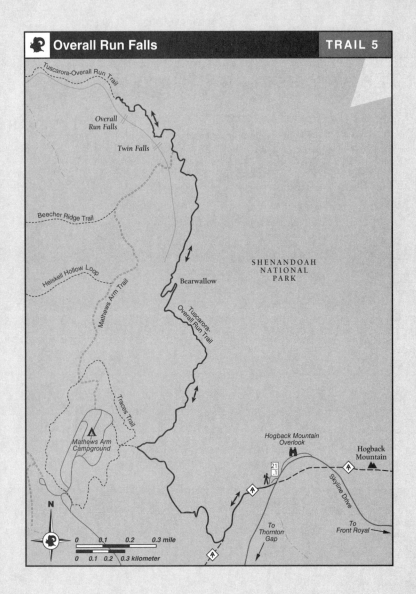

Overall Run Falls

TRAIL 5

Tuscarora-Overall Run Trail

Overall
Run Falls

Twin Falls

Beecher Ridge Trail

Heiskell Hollow Loop

Mathews Arm Trail

Bearwallow

Tuscarora-
Overall Run Trail

SHENANDOAH
NATIONAL
PARK

Traces Trail

Mathews Arm
Campground

Hogback Mountain
Overlook

Hogback
Mountain

21
1

Skyline Drive

N

0   0.1   0.2   0.3 mile

0   0.1   0.2   0.3 kilometer

To
Thornton
Gap

To
Front Royal

Overall Run Falls

This there-and-back hike holds great rewards when you arrive—the park's highest falls and a grand vista beyond—and a warm-up fall along the way. And the trek is not too hard either. Start with a pleasant mountaintop stroll on the Appalachian Trail, then wend your way down the slopes of Hogback Mountain, crossing many flats. Enter the Overall Run watershed. Pass Twin Falls, then come to Overall Run Falls. From a rocky precipice, you can see the nearby cataract and a whole lot more in the distance. Others will be enjoying the scenery with you, but it is not nearly as busy as Dark Hollow Falls and other cascades in the park's Central District. Nearby Mathews Arm Campground offers 217 campsites from May through October.

Best Time

Winter and early spring are the best times to see Shenandoah's highest falls. This locale also presents great views when the skies are clear, so keep that in mind.

Finding the Trail

The hike starts at the parking area just south of the Hogback Mountain Overlook, milepost 21.1 on Skyline Drive. To reach the trailhead from the Thornton Gap Entrance Station, take Skyline Drive north for 10.4 miles to the parking area on the west side of Skyline Drive, just before Hogback Mountain Overlook.

TRAIL USE
Dayhiking
LENGTH
6.8 miles, 4–5 hours
CUMULATIVE ELEVATION +/-
-1,500'/+1,500'
DIFFICULTY
– 1 2 3 **4** 5 +
TRAIL TYPE
Out & Back
START & FINISH
N38° 45.627'
W78° 16.953'

FEATURES
Ridgeline
Stream
Autumn Colors
Geologic Interest
Waterfall
Wildflowers
Wildlife
Great Views

FACILITIES
Campground nearby

Trail Description

Meet up with the Appalachian Trail (AT) as it skirts the south side of the parking area. ▶1 Turn right on the AT, heading southbound. Gently climb through lovely fern-carpeted woodland, passing a few rock outcrops. At a high point a spur leads left to jagged rocks and a limited view. Level off, then meet the Tuscarora-Overall Run Trail at 0.4 mile. ▶2 Turn right on the Tuscarora-Overall Run Trail. It proceeds downhill, snaking between rocks from which rise a rich forest. Rock and wood erosion bars cross the trail and form steps. Make a couple of switchbacks before coming to another trail junction at 1.1 miles. ▶3 Here, run into a connector to the Traces Nature Trail. You aren't far from Mathews Arm Campground.

Turn right, staying on the Tuscarora-Overall Run Trail. At 1.2 miles, pass a large embedded boulder on your left, then begin making your way down Hogback Mountain in stair-step fashion. The path will drop off, then level off, drop off again, and then level off once more. At 1.6 miles, step over the uppermost part of Overall Run. This trickling branch increases hope that there is a waterfall at the end of this thus far dry hike. These high-elevation flats seem to attract bears, which I have seen

 Ridgeline

 Autumn Colors

This trek leads to the park's tallest cataract.

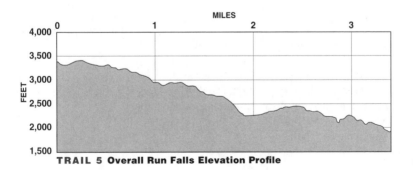

TRAIL 5 Overall Run Falls Elevation Profile

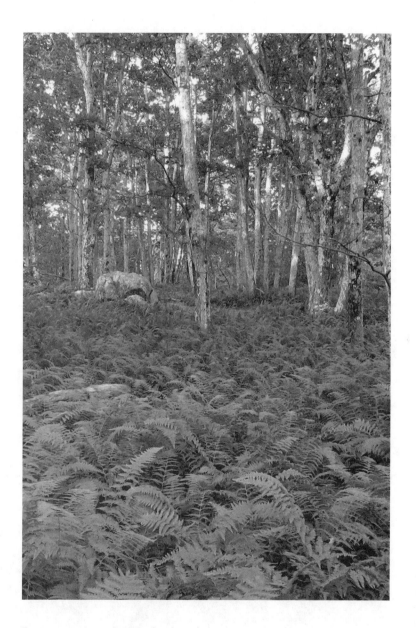

Fern-carpeted woodland *borders the trail.*

Wildlife

multiple times hereabouts. This area is shown on topo maps as "Bearwallow."

At 2.9 miles, the trail intersects the Mathews Arm Trail, which leaves left toward Mathews Arm Campground. Keep right. ▶4 Walk a short distance to another concrete signpost. Here, pass the now-abandoned section of Mathews Arm Trail. At this point you are likely wondering what water feeds the falls. The Tuscarora-Overall Run Trail answers the question, as you turn left down toward Overall Run on wood-and-earth steps. Reach the first cataract, Twin Falls, at 3.1 miles. ▶5

Stream

Wildflowers

Waterfall

A side trail leads left to the top of Twin Falls and a rock outcrop where you can view it. A large boulder splits Overall Run and divides the water, resulting in two streams dropping 29 feet. That is only the warm-up fall, but at least you are along and within earshot of moving water.

Keep astride the canyon, passing through laurel-oak woods. Tempting outcrops lure you to the edge of the valley, but they aren't *the* viewpoint. You will know it when you get there. Come to a wide open cliff at 3.4 miles. ▶6

Geologic Interest

Great Views

Waterfall

The world opens beyond. To your left tumbles Overall Run Falls, at 93 feet the park's highest. The cataract drops over a huge rock face into the gorge below. More rock forms a wall on the far side of the falls. Nearby, other outcrops form vantage spots. The Overall Run canyon plunges below. It's a long way down there! The canyon maw divulges Page Valley and Massanutten Mountain in the backdrop. In the distance rise the Alleghenies and West Virginia—a great view overall and one of my favorites in the park.

大 MILESTONES

▶1	0.0	Parking area at milepost 21.1
▶2	0.4	Right on Tuscarora-Overall Run Trail
▶3	1.1	Stay right on Tuscarora-Overall Run Trail
▶4	2.9	Mathews Arm Trail leaves left
▶5	3.1	Twin Falls
▶6	3.4	Overall Run Falls

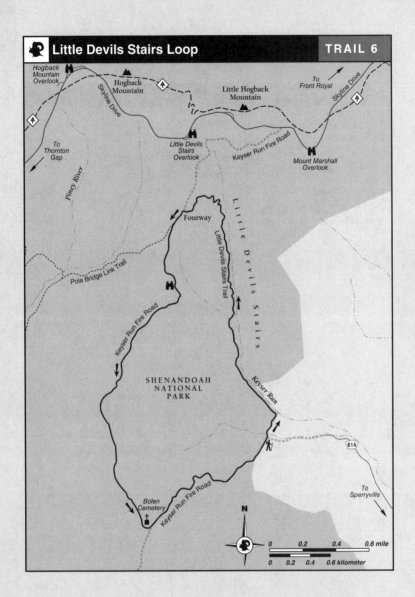

Little Devils Stairs Loop

TRAIL 6

Hogback Mountain Overlook

Hogback Mountain

Skyline Drive

Little Hogback Mountain

To Front Royal

Skyline Drive

To Thornton Gap

Little Devils Stairs Overlook

Keyser Run Fire Road

Mount Marshall Overlook

Piney River

Fourway

L i t t l e   D e v i l s   S t a i r s

Little Devils Stairs Trail

Pole Bridge Link Trail

Keyser Run Fire Road

SHENANDOAH
NATIONAL
PARK

Keyser Run

Keyser Run

614

Bolen Cemetery

Keyser Run Fire Road

To Sperryville

N

| 0 | 0.2 | 0.4 | 0.6 mile |

| 0 | 0.2 | 0.4 | 0.6 kilometer |

Little Devils Stairs Loop

This physically challenging but visually rewarding hike gives you something for every step you take. You undertake the challenging part (heading up Little Devils Stairs Canyon) at the beginning when you are fresh. The water, the rocks, the trees—there is beauty everywhere you look in this rough canyon. After emerging from the canyon, cruise down the mountains on Keyser Run Fire Road, taking in a well-earned vista and then passing pioneer internment Bolen Cemetery along the way.

Best Time

This hike requires multiple crossings of Keyser Run, at this point a smallish stream. Nonetheless, the crossings are easier from mid-spring beyond into early winter. When the leaves are off, you can fully appreciate the rocky gorge of Little Devils Stairs.

Finding the Trail

From Thornton Gap, take US 211 east for 7 miles to Sperryville. At a three-way intersection and the sign for the Sperryville Historic District, continue on US 211 east for 2.2 miles to VA 622, Gid Brown Hollow Road. Turn left on VA 622, and follow it for 1.9 miles to VA 614, Keyser Run Road. Turn left on VA 614, following it for 3.1 miles as it turns to gravel and ends at the Little Devils Stairs parking area. The Little Devils Stairs Trail leaves the right-hand side of the parking area.

TRAIL USE
Dayhiking, Backpacking

LENGTH
5.4 miles, 3½–4½ hours

CUMULATIVE ELEVATION +/-
+1,390'/-1,390'

DIFFICULTY
– 1 2 3 **4** 5 +

TRAIL TYPE
Loop

START & FINISH
N38° 43.838'
W78° 15.491'

FEATURES
Ridgeline
Stream
Geologic Interest
Wildflowers
Waterfall
Autumn Colors
Historic Interest
Great Views

FACILITIES
None

Trail Description

Leave the Little Devils Stairs parking area on the Little Devils Stairs Trail, and immediately step over two small streams. ▶1 Enter what once was a field in level woods. Notice the piles of rock, left over from when hardscrabble farmers squeezed out a life in this stony land.

At 0.2 mile reach a gap alongside Keyser Run, which cuts the Little Devils Stairs Canyon. Turn left and begin to trace the creek upstream. At this point the grade is gentle, as the canyon hasn't closed yet. The footing is rocky. Large boulders are strewn about the hardwoods that shade the trail.

At 0.6 mile, the canyon closes in. Look for more pioneer walls. It's amazing to think pre-park Virginians lived in this sloped, nothing-but-stone vale that contrasts mightily with the fertile lands of the nearby Shenandoah Valley. But most of the people who resided in these parts preferred the mountain way of life and the trials that came with it, including the labor involved in building these rock walls.

At 0.9 mile, cross Keyser Run on the first of many crossings, all of which should be simple rock-hops at normal water levels. ▶2 Given the nature of Shenandoah's streams, Keyser Run is more rock

Historic Interest

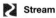

Stream

Wildflowers

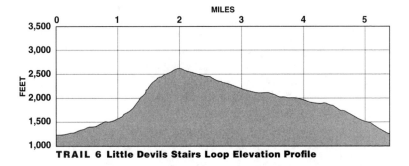

TRAIL 6 Little Devils Stairs Loop Elevation Profile

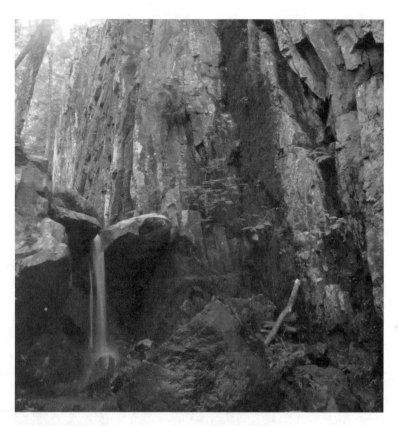

Keyser Run *spills between boulders against a sheer canyon wall backdrop.*

than water, and it often fans into braids that flow only during high-water events. The canyon narrows, and the forest of basswood, sycamore, and witch hazel becomes lush. Rock citadels rise to form canyon walls. Walk over, around, and among large boulders that litter the canyon floor. Beside you, the stream seeks its way down the gorge as fast as gravity allows.

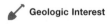
Geologic Interest

Trail and creek merge time and again. The steep gradient of the stream creates occasional pools harboring trout and other aquatic life. The sheer walls of the canyon rise straight up above you. In other places scree slopes descend to the trail's edge. Tall and straight tulip trees grow on the rocky soil where they can gain purchase. Stinging nettles spread across the canyon floor where they can settle. The trail is very steep here and sometimes hard to follow through the rock jumbles. Stone steps aid hikers in places, but you will likely find places where occasional floods have undermined them. Watch for the blue blazes and keep going up.

At 1.4 miles, just after a crossing to the right-hand bank, you hike past a slide cascade that ends in a trailside plunge pool. The trail steepens. At mile 1.6, make your last crossing of Keyser Run, ending up on the left side of the gorge. ▶3 Gently climb a series of switchbacks and level off, meeting the Keyser Run Fire Road at 2.0 miles. You have just climbed 1,500 feet. This trail junction is known as Fourway.

Turn left on the Keyser Run Fire Road, and begin a trifling descent after your rigorous climb through the rigorous canyon. ▶4 Trailside hardwoods only partially canopy the track. Enjoy the forest around you, breathing easy. Funny thing about the fire road: It was once known as Jinney Gray Fire Road, but after her history was lost to time, the park service changed the name to Keyser Run Fire Road. In summer wildflowers color the edges of the track in summer, and ripe berries tempt the hiker.

At 2.5 miles, a spur trail leads left to a rock outcrop and vista. ▶5 Here, you can look into the canyon below as well as out at waves of mountains beyond and the crest of the Blue Ridge. Watch for a small rocked-in spring branch at 3.1 miles. At other times, small seeps spill over the trail. Pass under a transmission line at 3.8 miles. Enter a deep woods flat dominated by white pine and some large-for-the-species sassafras trees. Watch for rock fence lines and larger trees of old homesites.

Autumn Colors

Waterfall

Hike up a boulder-strewn canyon resembling the American West.

Great Views

Arrive at Bolen Cemetery at 4.3 miles. The well-tended internment is lined with maples and surrounded by a rock wall. The graves range from carved marble to simple fieldstones. Just beyond, the Hull School Trail leaves right. Stay left on Keyser Run Fire Road, and descend beneath more white pines. ▶6 Watch for more rock walls and the old pre-park road running parallel to the modern fire road. Pass around a pole gate at 5.2 miles. Keep left, and complete your loop at mile 5.4. ▶7

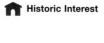 **Historic Interest**

🚶	**MILESTONES**	
▶1	0.0	Little Devils Stairs Trailhead
▶2	0.9	First crossing of Keyser Run
▶3	1.6	Last crossing of Keyser Run
▶4	2.2	Left on Keyser Run Fire Road
▶5	2.5	Vista
▶6	4.3	Left just after Bolen Cemetery
▶7	5.4	Little Devils Stairs Trailhead

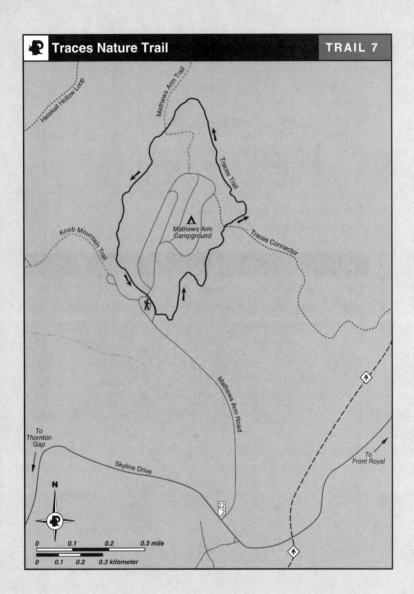

Traces Nature Trail

Sometimes we forget that this wonderful national park open to everyone was once the home of many a Virginian. As Shenandoah National Park was being realized, residents within these boundaries were bought out and had to move elsewhere. Upon the park's establishment more than 400 families comprised of more than 2,000 citizens still resided in Shenandoah. Some were fighting the forced sale of their lands, while others, some squatters, simply didn't have the means to move on. Still others wanted to live out their lives in the mountains that they loved.

Eventually the Resettlement Administration (an arm of the federal government) stepped in and made plots available in the adjacent lowlands that the former Shenandoah residents could purchase on favorable terms. A few pioneers arranged lifetime leases, allowing them to live in the park until they passed away. The last living park resident called Shenandoah home until 1975.

Today, careful observation in many areas of the park will reveal traces of the pioneer settlements—rock walls, building foundations, broken crockery shards, a rusted washtub, and exotic flowers and bushes that still bloom every spring. The changes in land use from residential to park are especially striking here on the Traces Nature Trail. Where once Virginians made a life, we have a recreational path that wanders through high-country woods, encircling a campground used by modern visitors who come to these soothing Potomac Highlands seeking a respite from the hurries of everyday urban life.

Note: Pets are prohibited on this trail.

TRAIL USE
Dayhiking,
Child-Friendly,
Pets Prohibited

LENGTH
1.6 miles, 1–2 hours

CUMULATIVE ELEVATION +/-
+215'/-215'

DIFFICULTY
– 1 **2** 3 4 5 +

TRAIL TYPE
Loop

START & FINISH
N38° 45.604'
W78° 17.871'

FEATURES
Ridgeline
Autumn Colors
Historic Interest
Camping

FACILITIES
Campground nearby

Best Time

This short family hike is best done when Mathews Arm Campground is open, generally mid-May through October. Otherwise you have to walk the campground access road from Skyline Drive to get to the trail.

Finding the Trail

From milepost 22.2 on Skyline Drive, follow the entrance road from Skyline Drive into Mathews Arm Campground for 0.6 mile, reaching a T-intersection just after the campground entrance station. Turn right here, then immediately turn right again into a large parking area. The Traces Nature Trail starts at the far end of the parking lot.

Trail Description

Leave the large parking area on the marked Traces Nature Trail on a rocky path. ▶1 (Don't take the wide track leading to the campground amphitheater.) Start at 2,700 feet, which makes for a decidedly cooler climate than the Shenandoah Valley below. It isn't long before you find your first

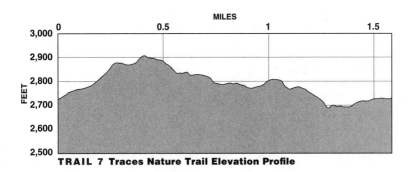

TRAIL 7 Traces Nature Trail Elevation Profile

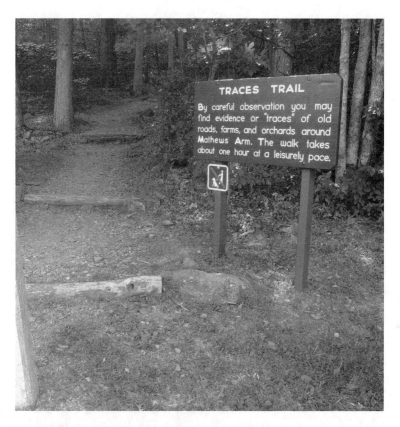

The first few *steps of the Traces Nature Trail*

"trace" of pre-park settlement, as the trail veers left, joining an old roadbed. Oaks, birch, and witch hazel rise above a forest floor of fern and stone. The term *road* conjures up cars, but this track was more likely used by horses, wagons—and feet.

 Autumn Colors

At 0.3 mile, come to a rock outcrop and leveled area, perhaps a homesite, though the terrain looks inhospitable. But near the trail you can see the telltale rock walls, erected through backbreaking exertion and likely to be here long after many of our modern buildings have fallen by the wayside. The

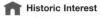 **Historic Interest**

walls were built to simply remove stones from fields or to keep critters from getting into the garden or grazing in the front yard. Farm animals generally roamed at will and were rounded up when the time came for slaughtering. Typically, settlers would notch the ears of critters to identify ownership. Today, deer roam the area.

At 0.5 mile, reach an intersection. Stay left with the Traces Trail, ▶2 but look how a line of trees borders the trail going straight. Imagine a clearing, yard, and home in this locale. Moving forward, you enter a younger forest—it was likely a field when the park was established. It is estimated that more than a third of the park was open country in 1935, when the park came to be. Descend past more rock walls, then cross a spring seep. Springs were crucial for locating highland homesteads like those found on Mathews Arm.

Continue cruising below the campground. Partial views open to the east as the terrain steepens. Pass boulder outcrops—these were impediments to pre-park residents, yet they are sought out today, especially the outcrops that avail far-reaching vistas. Intersect the wide Mathews Arm Trail at 1.0 mile. ▶3 Keep straight here, still on the Traces Nature Trail. The campground is but 0.1 mile distant. Bigger trees rise here. Outcrops to the right of the path provide partial views toward the Shenandoah Valley to the west. Before you know it the hike is over at 1.6 miles. ▶4

While in the vicinity, consider adding a stay at Mathews Arm Campground. You can overnight here on a first-come, first-served basis, but reservations are available on one loop. Each campsite has a picnic table and fire grate. Water spigots, restrooms, and recycling centers are situated throughout the three loops of the campground. Most of the sites are shaded, though a few have a mix of sun and shade. There are some pull-through sites for camper rigs.

During the week sites are almost always available. The higher elevation keeps it a good 10 degrees cooler than the Shenandoah Valley below. Make sure and store your food carefully, since Mathews Arm is bear country.

🚶	**MILESTONES**	
▶1	0.0	Traces Nature Trail parking
▶2	0.5	Stay left with Traces Nature Trail at signpost
▶3	1.0	Cross Mathews Arm Trail
▶4	1.6	Campground access road near parking area

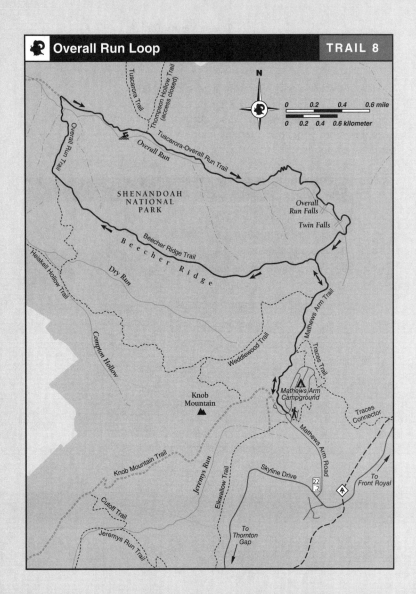

Overall Run Loop

TRAIL 8

N

0	0.2 0.4 0.6 mile
0	0.2 0.4 0.6 kilometer

Tuscarora Trail

Thompson Hollow Trail (access closed)

Overall Run Trail

Tuscarora-Overall Run Trail

Overall Run

SHENANDOAH NATIONAL PARK

Overall Run Falls

Twin Falls

Beecher Ridge Trail

B e e c h e r   R i d g e

Heiskell Hollow Trail

Dry Run

Mathews Arm Trail

Compton Hollow

Weddlewood Trail

Traces Trail

Mathews Arm Campground

Traces Connector

Knob Mountain

Knob Mountain Trail

Jeremys Run

Elkwallow Trail

Mathews Arm Road

Skyline Drive

To Front Royal

Cutoff Trail

22
2

To Thornton Gap

Jeremys Run Trail

Overall Run Loop

Leave the kids behind on this challenging loop that is a personal favorite. Beyond its high point near Mathews Arm Campground, the hike drops more than 2,000 feet, and then climbs back up, every foot. Leave near the Mathews Arm Campground entrance station. Circle the campground before joining remote Beecher Ridge, making a glorious walk through lush forests and parklike woodlands before dropping to Overall Run. The lower part of Overall Run reveals its former pioneer presence. Work upstream in a rugged gorge, passing a superlative swimming hole. The gorge tightens and narrows, and the stream is forced to drop over a series of falls into more large pools. Come to Overall Run Falls, the park's highest at 93 feet. You can observe this cataract and enjoy a mountain panorama before making your way back to the trailhead.

Best Time

This hike is best done when nearby Mathews Arm Campground is open, generally mid-May through October. Otherwise you have to walk the campground access road from Skyline Drive to get to the trail. The crossings of Overall Run will be easier then as well.

Finding the Trail

From milepost 22.2 on Skyline Drive, follow the entrance road from Skyline Drive into Mathews Arm Campground for 0.6 mile, reaching a T-intersection just after the campground entrance station. Turn

TRAIL USE
Dayhiking, Backpacking
LENGTH
9.2 miles, 5½–7 hours
CUMULATIVE ELEVATION +/-
-2,060'/+2,060'
DIFFICULTY
– 1 2 3 4 **5** +
TRAIL TYPE
Loop
START & FINISH
N38° 45.640'
W78° 17.899'

FEATURES
Stream
Wildlife
Autumn Colors
Waterfall
Secluded
Historic Interest
Geologic Interest
Swimming
Steep
Great Views

FACILITIES
Campground nearby

right here, then immediately turn right again into a large parking area.

Trail Description

The Traces Nature Trail has two entrances from the trailhead parking area. Make sure and pick up the Traces Nature Trail that leaves from the T-intersection near the campground entrance station rather than the one that leads directly from the trailhead parking area near the campground amphitheater. ▶1 On the proper segment of the Traces Nature Trail, you immediately pass under a power line, then roll in rocky highland woods.

Meet the Mathews Arm Trail at 0.6 mile. ▶2 Turn left here on a wide, roadlike track, descending to pass a closing meadow on your right. Look for deer here; you may well see one in the morning or evening. Pass the Weddlewood Trail at 0.9 mile. The wide roadbed makes for easy walking, but the Mathews Arm Trail soon narrows to meet the Beecher Ridge Trail at 1.4 miles. Turn left here, joining this solitude-soaked path. ▶3 Enter a remote section of the park. Single-track Beecher Ridge Trail descends in oak-dominated woods. The valley of Overall Run falls away to your right. This trail is heavily traveled by bears—you will likely see bear

This hike has it all, including distance and elevation challenges.

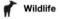 **Wildlife**

▲ **Ridgeline**

 Secluded

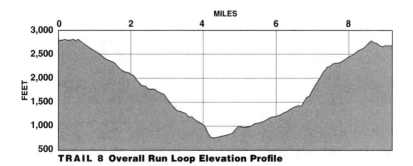

TRAIL 8 Overall Run Loop Elevation Profile

scat on the path in summer. Join the crest of wide Beecher Ridge at 2.2 miles. Level off in parklike woodland at 2.4 miles. Enjoy the forest cruise as you skim an inconsequential knob. Notice the still-standing locust trees here—many are beginning to fall in inevitable forest succession. Hickories and oaks, shaded by the locusts, are taking over, and the locust trees, notoriously rot-resistant, will eventually decay back into the earth, feeding the future mighty oaks and hickories.

🍁 **Autumn Colors**

Resume a rapid descent amid oak-laden rocky woods with little ground cover. The ridgeline narrows. Pines join the fray before making a trail junction at 3.7 miles. Turn toward Overall Run on the Beecher-Overall Connector Trail. ►4 You, however, keep forward, curving north on a dry ridge widespread with blueberry bushes. The woods thicken when you enter the Overall Run valley. Reach Overall Run at 4.2 miles. ►5 Here, the stream is braided and is more rock than water, perhaps even entirely dry, in summer and fall. Following rains it can be torrential. If it is, do not attempt to cross it. Continue stepping across several stream braids, making the north side of the run.

At 4.3 miles, turn right here at a concrete marker post, joining an old roadbed heading easterly, officially on the Tuscarora-Overall Trail. Note the rock walls in this wide valley, evidence of former settlements and hardscrabble farming in this stony soil, now supporting white pines.

🏠 **Historic Interest**

Buckled rock walls constrict the valley at 4.8 miles. In high water the whole stream funnels through this portal.

🜨 **Stream**

The trail climbs away from the stream, and at 4.9 miles, you reach a potentially confusing four-way junction. ►6 To your left is a campsite. The blue-blazed Tuscarora-Overall Run Trail keeps straight, and to your right, a trail leads to a sunny outcrop and a surprisingly deep swimming hole

Swimming

below a rock slab cascade. This is a special area. Please treat it with care. The open outcrop is great for drying off after a dip in the crystalline pool. The hike continues climbing to shortly meet the Thompson Hollow Trail, which leads left to the park boundary. ▶7 Access is currently closed.

Keep making your way up the scenic gorge, pocked with spicebush and pawpaw, on a very rocky track that slows your progress. Cross Overall Run at 5.6 and 6.0 miles. The trail becomes very steep as you leave the creek at 6.3 miles, switchbacking toward the canyon rim. ▶8 At 6.6 miles, a spur trail leads right to a cliff that many hikers

Steep

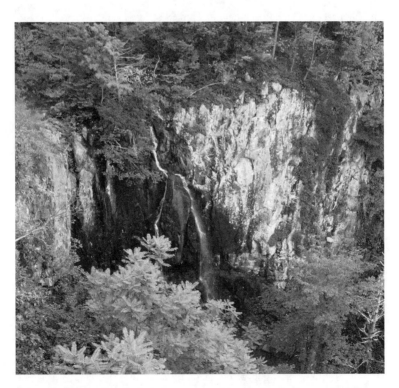

Overall Run Falls, *the park's highest cataract at 93 feet, also goes by the name Big Falls.*

bypass. ▶9 You can look up toward an outcrop you will soon be standing on. Make the rim and reach another cliff with a fantastic view at 7.2 miles. ▶10 Across the gorge is Overall Run Falls, the park's highest at 93 feet. In winter, the fall may be frozen over the entire rock face. In summer, flow can be low and sluggish. Below, Overall Run Canyon winds its way toward the Page Valley. Beyond stands Massanutten Mountain. Beyond that rise the Alleghenies.

Continue up the rim, and soon pass wooded Twin Falls to your right, a much smaller drop at 29 feet. You have to go off the trail a little to get a good view. The path switchbacks away from the creek and comes to a concrete post and the Mathews Arm Trail at 7.4 miles. Stay right here and just ahead the Tuscarora-Overall Run Trail leaves left for the AT. ▶11 Stay right with the Mathews Arm Trail, making a gentle uptick to reach the Beecher Ridge Trail at 7.8 miles. ▶12 From here, make a 1.4-mile backtrack to the trailhead. ▶13

Geologic Interest

Waterfall

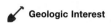
Great Views

Waterfall

🚶	**MILESTONES**	
▶1	0.0	Traces Nature Trail parking
▶2	0.6	Left on Mathews Arm Trail
▶3	1.4	Left on Beecher Ridge Trail
▶4	3.7	Right on Beecher-Overall Connector Trail
▶5	4.2	Right on Tuscarora-Overall Run Trail after crossing Overall Run
▶6	4.9	Swimming hole on right
▶7	5.0	Thompson Hollow Trail leaves left
▶8	6.3	Leave creek
▶9	6.6	Spur to cliff
▶10	7.2	Overall Run Falls and Page Valley vista
▶11	7.4	Right with Mathews Arm Trail
▶12	7.8	Pass Beecher Ridge Trail
▶13	9.2	Traces Nature Trail parking

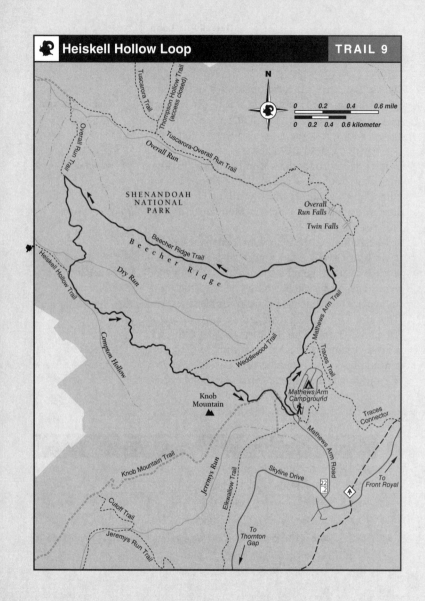

Heiskell Hollow Loop

This hike explores the least visited ridge and valley of the greater Mathews Arm area of the park, and is one of the least hiked quality circuits in the park. It has no single superlative feature to draw hikers in but offers you a chance to explore the park in solitude. First, circle around Mathews Arm Campground on the Traces Nature Trail, eventually reaching secluded Beecher Ridge. Travel the spine of this regally forested highland before picking up the Heiskell Hollow Trail. Dip into the East Fork Valley before winding your way up Keyser Hollow and back onto Mathews Arm. Plenty of pioneer evidence awaits a sharp-eyed hiker.

Best Time

This hike is best done when nearby Mathews Arm Campground is open, generally mid-May through October. Otherwise you have to walk the campground access road from Skyline Drive to get to the trail.

Finding the Trail

From milepost 22.2 on Skyline Drive, follow the entrance road from Skyline Drive into Mathews Arm Campground for 0.6 mile, reaching a T-intersection just after the campground entrance station. Turn right here, then immediately turn right again into a large parking area.

TRAIL USE
Dayhiking, Backpacking

LENGTH
7.2 miles, 4–5 hours

CUMULATIVE ELEVATION +/-
-1,620'/+1,620'

DIFFICULTY
– 1 2 3 **4** 5 +

TRAIL TYPE
Loop

START & FINISH
N38° 45.640'
W78° 17.899'

FEATURES
Ridgeline
Stream
Autumn Colors
Wildflowers
Secluded
Wildlife
Historic Interest

FACILITIES
Campground nearby

Trail Description

Start your loop on the Traces Nature Trail. ▶1 Be careful because it has two entrances from the trailhead parking area. Make sure and pick up the Traces Nature Trail that leaves from the T-intersection near the campground entrance station rather than the one that leads directly from the trailhead parking area near the campground amphitheater. Once you are on the proper segment of the Traces Nature Trail, you immediately pass under a power line, then undulate in rocky highland woods.

Come to Mathews Arm Trail at 0.6 mile. Turn left here. ▶2 Pass a small field where deer may be seen browsing. The Weddlewood Trail leaves left at 0.9 mile. Keep straight on the wide Mathews Arm Trail. The wide roadbed makes for easy walking, but the Mathews Arm Trail narrows before coming to Beecher Ridge Trail at 1.4 miles. Turn left here. ▶3 The faint, but clear trail attests to the solitude found along its length. Tall oaks shade single-track Beecher Ridge Trail. The valley of Overall Run falls away to your right and East Fork to your left. It seems bears use the trail more than people—you will likely see bear scat on the path in summer.

Join the crest of wide Beecher Ridge at 2.2 miles. Level off in parklike woodland at 2.4 miles. Resume a rapid descent amid oak-laden rocky woods with

Solitude lovers will enjoy this circuit.

🦌 **Wildlife**

▲ **Ridgeline**

👤 **Secluded**

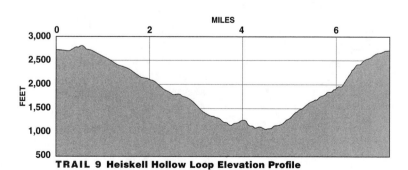

TRAIL 9 Heiskell Hollow Loop Elevation Profile

little ground cover. The ridgeline narrows. Pines mix in with the oaks.

Come to a forlorn trail junction at 3.7 miles. ►4 Turn left here onto Heiskell Hollow. Wander southeasterly through pine-oak woods. Watch for old pioneer roads crossing Heiskell Hollow Trail. Dip to a dry streambed, climb a bit, then resume your quest for East Fork. Reach East Fork at 4.4 miles. Traverse a rocky area dividing East Fork from Moody Creek, coming to the Heiskell Hollow Trail at 4.5 miles. ►5 Turn left here, ascending along Moody Creek in Keyser Hollow. Angle up a mountainside in piney woods with a grassy understory. Meet the Weddlewood Trail at 6.2 miles. ►6

Stay with Heiskell Hollow Trail, ascending through open, rock-strewn forest escorted by rock walls. Watch for old roads splintering off the path. Also look for large oaks, which have grown tall above the rocky floor. Emerge onto the crumbling asphalt of the access road for Mathews Arm water treatment station at 6.8 miles. Turn left, ascending a wide track. ►7 Come out near Mathews Arm Campground entrance station at 7.2 miles, completing your loop. ►8

Secluded

Stream

Wildflowers

Historic Interest

🚶	**MILESTONES**	
►1	0.0	Traces Nature Trail parking
►2	0.6	Left on Mathews Arm Trail
►3	1.4	Left on Beecher Ridge Trail
►4	3.7	Stay left at intersection, still on Beecher Ridge Trail
►5	4.5	Left on Heiskell Hollow Trail
►6	6.2	Pass Weddlewood Trail
►7	6.8	Left on crumbling asphalt road
►8	7.2	Mathews Arm Campground

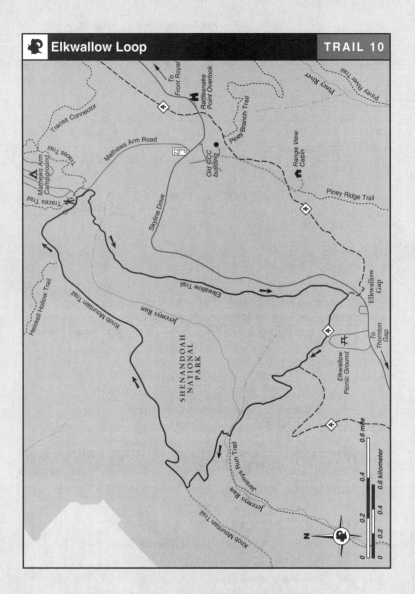

Elkwallow Loop

TRAIL 10

To Front Royal

Rattlesnake Point Overlook

Piney River Trail

Piney River

Traces Connector

Mathews Arm Road

Piney Branch Trail

Range View Cabin

Mathews Arm Campground

Traces Trail

Old CCC building

Piney Ridge Trail

Skyline Drive

Traces Trail

Heiskell Hollow Trail

Knob Mountain Trail

Elkwallow Trail

Jeremys Run

Elkwallow Gap

To Thornton Gap

SHENANDOAH NATIONAL PARK

Elkwallow Picnic Ground

Jeremys Run Trail

Jeremys Run

Knob Mountain Trail

0.6 mile

0.6 kilometer

0.4

0.2

0.4

0.2

0

0

N

Elkwallow Loop

It's a wonder that this classic Shenandoah circuit hike isn't done more, considering the proximity of camping and other national park facilities to the often-level loop. First, leave the Mathews Arm Campground on the Elkwallow Trail. It navigates boulders galore before settling down and making a pleasantly level highland track on the west side of the Blue Ridge. The loop joins the Appalachian Trail near Elkwallow Wayside, where food and other supplies are available. Pass a picnic area and spring before joining Jeremys Run Trail, dipping to Jeremys Run. Cross the fine mountain stream then climb a stony slope, joining the seldom-trod Knob Mountain Trail. This path offers everywhere-you-look beauty on a remarkably level track, allowing you to enjoy the national park scenery. The final ascent leads back to Mathews Arm Campground.

Best Time

This hike is best done when Mathews Arm Campground is open, generally mid-May through October. Otherwise you have to walk the campground access road from Skyline Drive to get to the trail.

Finding the Trail

From milepost 22.2 on Skyline Drive, follow the entrance road from Skyline Drive into Mathews Arm Campground for 0.6 mile, reaching a T-intersection just after the campground entrance station. Turn right here, then immediately turn right again into a

TRAIL USE
Dayhiking

LENGTH
5.6 miles, 3–4 hours

CUMULATIVE
ELEVATION +/-
-825'/-825'

DIFFICULTY
– 1 2 **3** 4 5 +

TRAIL TYPE
Loop

START & FINISH
N38° 45.604'
W78° 17.871'

FEATURES
Ridgeline
Stream
Autumn Colors
Wildflowers
Wildlife
Secluded

FACILITIES
Campground and
   camp store
Picnic area

large parking area. The Elkwallow Trail starts across the campground access road from the parking area, near the entrance station (Driving in, you can see the Elkwallow Trail on your left, just before coming to the campground entrance station).

Trail Description

Join the Elkwallow Trail ►1 as it briefly follows a grassy road then splits right as a single-track path heading downhill in a rocky hardwood forest of witch hazel, white oak, and fire cherry. Drop off a stone bluff to reach a high-elevation wetland. A long boardwalk, rare for this mountain park, spans these headwaters of Jeremys Run. Continue on the level as Jeremys Run falls away below. This easy walking allows you to observe the forest comprehensively. The woodlands of Shenandoah National Park have been in a near continual state of change since the park's inception. First, the cleared pastures of pre-park settlers began the slow process of succession from field to forest. Later, the gypsy moth came in and decimated the mighty oaks of Shenandoah, setting off another chain reaction of reforestation where the oaks fell. Lately, the demise of the hemlock has shaped the woodland. Once again

 Wildflowers

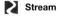 Stream

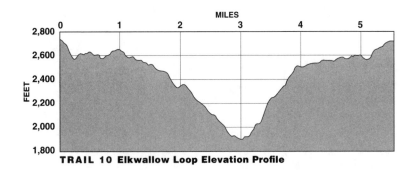

TRAIL 10 Elkwallow Loop Elevation Profile

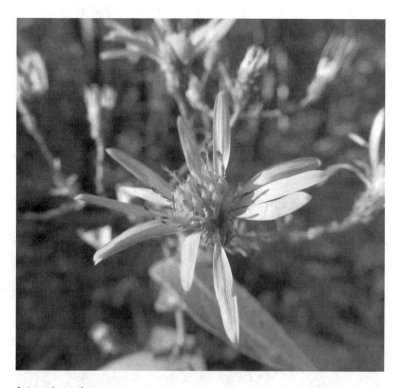

Asters *glow in the autumn sun.*

opportunistic plants are coming in and rising where hemlocks once stood.

In winter views open to your right. Pass an obvious trailside boulder at 1.2 miles. The next mile or so is a good place to spot deer. The open forest and adjacent clearings lure them in. Come near Skyline Drive, then intersect the Appalachian Trail (AT) at 1.8 miles. Turn right here, ▶2 southbound on Shenandoah's master path. (Elkwallow Wayside is just ahead if you keep straight on the Elkwallow Trail. The Wayside offers drinks, food, and other supplies in season.) The AT meanders downhill in slightly-sloped forest with little understory. At 2.1 miles, turn right with the AT, as a spur trail leads left

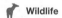 **Wildlife**

to Elkwallow Picnic Ground. ▶3 Soon pass a spring used by AT hikers, where the long dismantled Elkwallow Shelter once stood.

At 2.3 miles, leave the Appalachian Trail, joining the Jeremys Run Trail. ▶4 Work downhill entering the Jeremys Run Valley. Come to Jeremys Run and a trail intersection at 3.0 miles. Turn right here on the Knob Mountain Cutoff Trail to immediately walk across clear Jeremys Run on stones. Now comes the only hard part of the hike—a 350-foot climb in a half mile. Angle up the south slope of Knob Mountain. ▶5 Pass several partially open stone slabs on your switchback ascent amid hickories.

🌼 **Wildflowers**

📍 **Stream**

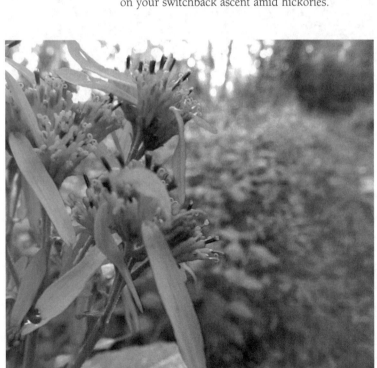

Trailside flowers *add fragrant beauty to fall.*

At 3.6 miles, turn right onto the Knob Mountain Trail, making another, milder climb on a wide track. ▶6 Level off at 3.9 miles, then make a glorious ridgeline walk. Sturdy white oaks and white pines shade the path. Watch for bears in the flats. Rocks have been cleared from the remarkably flat trail.

At 5.1 miles, reach a service road for the campground water treatment plant. Turn right on the crumbly asphalt, toward the campground. ▶7 Soon pass the Heiskell Hollow Trail. Ahead, pass around a chain gate, and emerge on blacktop near the campground entrance station, completing your hike at 5.6 miles. ▶8

Secluded

Ridgeline

Wildlife

🚶	**MILESTONES**	
▶1	0.0	Elkwallow Trailhead near Mathews Arm entrance station
▶2	1.8	Right on Appalachian Trail
▶3	2.1	Spur leads left to Elkwallow Picnic Ground
▶4	2.3	Right on Jeremys Run Trail
▶5	3.1	Right on Knob Mountain Cutoff Trail
▶6	3.6	Right on Knob Mountain Trail
▶7	5.1	Right on asphalt service road
▶8	5.6	End of hike near campground entrance station

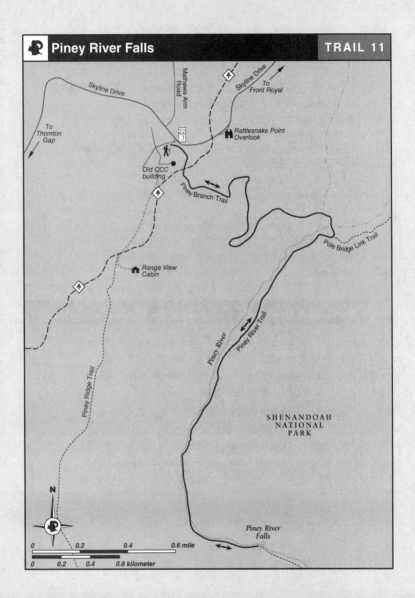

Skyline Drive

Mathews Arm Road

Skyline Drive
To Front Royal

To Thornton Gap

22
.1

Rattlesnake Point Overlook

Old CCC building

Piney Branch Trail

Range View Cabin

Pole Bridge Link Trail

Piney River

Piney River Trail

Piney Ridge Trail

SHENANDOAH NATIONAL PARK

N

Piney River Falls

0   0.2   0.4   0.6 mile

0   0.2 0.4   0.6 kilometer

Piney River Falls

It's surprising that this hike isn't more popular. The scenery along the way meets high Shenandoah standards, and the falls are a worthy destination. To get there, leave the high country, and gently wind your way through eye-pleasing, high-country woods. Work your way down through the Piney River Valley on old roads, and take a short side trail to the three-tier falls. It's a good way to spend an afternoon.

Best Time

The lesser-visited destination offers solitude most of the year. In spring it offers a bold watercourse and wildflowers. Summer is cool along the river. Fall has color. If you want maximum solitude, take this hike in winter.

Finding the Trail

From the Thornton Gap Entrance Station, take Skyline Drive north for 9.4 miles to the old Civilian Conservation Corps (CCC) building in the upper Piney River area. The entrance road is on your right at milepost 22.1, just north of the turn to Mathews Arm Campground on the left. Park in the designated visitor parking area across from the CCC building. The Piney Branch Trail starts between the parking area and Skyline Drive.

TRAIL USE
Dayhiking, Backpacking
LENGTH
6.8 miles, 3½–4½ hours
CUMULATIVE
ELEVATION +/-
-1,325'/+1,325'
DIFFICULTY
– 1 2 3 **4** 5 +
TRAIL TYPE
Out & Back
START & FINISH
N38° 45.037'
W78° 17.599'

FEATURES
Ridgeline
Stream
Waterfall
Wildflowers
Autumn Colors
Secluded

FACILITIES
None

Trail Description

▲ Ridgeline

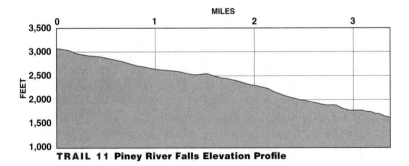 Stream

Start your hike at the back of the field between Skyline Drive and the parking area across from the old CCC camp building. ►1 Look for the concrete post marked "Piney Branch Trail." Begin walking through a forest of black locust trees in the process of taking over an old pasture. Up to a third of the land within the park was once field, pasture, or meadow—treeless. Even now the trees continue to inexorably reclaim former farm country, which was once woods even farther back in time. At 0.1 mile intersect the Appalachian Trail (AT) and continue straight on a track much fainter than the AT. Just ahead, cross a once grassy lane now growing up with trees. Note the apple trees in the area.

The Piney Branch Trail winds its way down to the valley, making very gentle, loping switchbacks. Pass by an open rock slab at 0.4 mile, then a wooded boulder field. The forest is much taller here than it is near the trailhead. The old roadbed comes to the upper reaches of the Piney River at mile 1.3. ►2 Big boulders line the small river. The grassy area beside the stream makes for a good place to relax. Curve right away from Piney River, crossing spring branches flowing between rocks. Park personnel did an outstanding job designing a

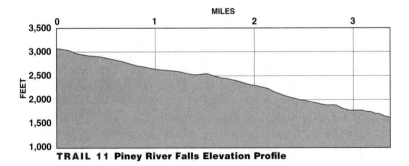

TRAIL 11 Piney River Falls Elevation Profile

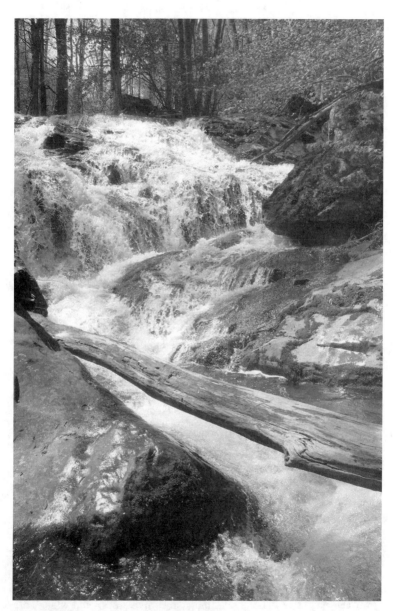

Piney River Falls *fans out over a rock face before slowing in a pool.*

Secluded

Wildflowers

Stream

Waterfall

dry track through this mushy area. The trail meets the Pole Bridge Link Trail at 1.5 miles. ►3

Turn right, staying with the now-narrower and even less-used section of the Piney Branch Trail. Wildflowers thrive in the Piney River Valley. The mountain laurel–lined path follows an old road on a slight downgrade. The gorge of Piney River cuts ever deeper to your right. At mile 2.0, the old road continues straight, but the Piney Branch Trail veers right and follows another old road. The trail runs a fair distance above the creek, descending at a moderate but steady clip.

At 2.7 miles, the trail comes very close to Piney River. ►4 A spur trail leads right to the riverside and a nice picnic spot. Continue along the waterway, appreciating its pools and shoals, in a wildflower-filled flat, where big boulders pock the rising hillside.

Cross the Piney River at 3.0 miles. ►5 This is a rock-hop at normal flows, but it takes a little footwork. Another method is to shed your shoes and socks and walk through the water with a stout stick as an aid. At lower levels this crossing is a breeze. You are now on the southern side of the river, and the falls are only 0.4 mile away. Watch and listen for other cascades along Piney River while making your way downstream. Cove hardwoods of yellow birch, black birch, red maple, and basswood shade the frothing watercourse.

Stumble through river rubble, rocks strewn here from high-water events. Ferns spread wide beside rock outcrops. Sycamores find their place amid the rocks and water. Pass two house-sized rock bluffs on your right at mile 3.2 in this rugged gorge. A hard-to-reach falls spills to your left. Begin listening for Piney River Falls, only 0.2 mile away. At mile 3.4, turn left on a side trail leading to the cataract. ►6 Piney River Falls is a 25-foot, tiered cascade that flows over mossy rock into a deep and wide pool.

Rock slabs border much of the drop and make for
good observation locales. It's a good place to cool off
after a hot hike. Relax a spell.

🚶	**MILESTONES**	
▶1	0.0	Old CCC building at milepost 22.1
▶2	1.3	Cross Piney River
▶3	1.5	Stay right with Piney Branch Trail
▶4	2.7	Come back along Piney River
▶5	3.0	Cross Piney River
▶6	3.4	Piney River Falls

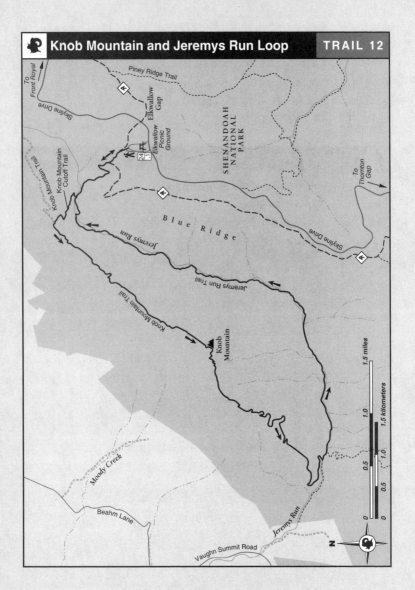

Knob Mountain and Jeremys Run Loop

TRAIL 12

To Front Royal

Skyline Drive

Piney Ridge Trail

Elkwallow Gap

Elkwallow Picnic Ground

SHENANDOAH NATIONAL PARK

To Thornton Gap

Knob Mountain Trail

Knob Mountain Cutoff Trail

Blue Ridge

Jeremys Run

Skyline Drive

Jeremys Run Trail

Knob Mountain Trail

Knob Mountain

1.5 miles

1.0

0.5

0

1.5 kilometers

1.0

0.5

0

Moody Creek

Beahm Lane

Jeremys Run

Vaughn Summit Road

N

Knob Mountain and Jeremys Run Loop

This is a long and yet rewarding loop exploring points high and low. Leave Elkwallow Picnic Ground (which has water, restrooms, and shaded tables), dropping to upper Jeremys Run, one of the park's biggest, wildest valleys. Climb to Knob Mountain, then traverse its ridgeline, enjoying views on the way to Jeremys Run. Make your way up gorgeous Jeremys Run valley, crossing the stream more than a dozen times. Watch for brook trout in the deep pools of Jeremys Run. You may want to cool off in the stream while down there. Leave the valley, backtracking to Elkwallow. Don't expect to have company on Knob Mountain, though you may see a few people along Jeremys Run.

Best Time

This is a great summertime hike. You can cruise the high country, and just when things get a little hot, the trek takes you along the pools of Jeremys Run, ideal for fishing or swimming. Fall is good too, since the low stream will make the 16 crossings easier. Conversely, the water may be too high during winter and early spring.

Finding the Trail

From Thornton Gap, take Skyline Drive north for 7.4 miles to Elkwallow Picnic Ground at milepost 24.1. Drive to the low end of the picnic area and park. The spur trail to the Appalachian Trail (AT) leaves here. The Elkwallow Wayside, a short distance north on Skyline Drive, has a camp store and

TRAIL USE
Dayhiking, Backpacking

LENGTH
13.1 miles,
8½–9½ hours

CUMULATIVE
ELEVATION +/-
-1,770'/+1,770'

DIFFICULTY
– 1 2 3 4 **5** +

TRAIL TYPE
Loop

START & FINISH
N38° 45.715'
W78° 18.295'

FEATURES
Stream
Ridgeline
Summit
Geologic Interest
Wildlife
Autumn Colors
Waterfall
Great Views
Camping
Swimming
Secluded
Steep

FACILITIES
Picnic area with water
    and restrooms
Camp store (in season)

food offerings during the warm season if you don't feel like picnicking.

Trail Description

This hike presents streamside and mountaintop highlights.

Start your loop on the spur trail leaving Elkwallow Picnic Ground. ▶1 Leave Elkwallow, and in fifty yards intersect the AT. Stay left, heading downhill, southbound through woods. Pass a marked spring on your left that serves up chilly water even on the hottest summer day. Meet the Jeremys Run Trail at 0.2 mile. ▶2 Keep straight on the Jeremys Run Trail, as the AT makes a hard left here. Travel a long abandoned roadbed on surprisingly level terrain. Shortly switchback downhill, crossing the outflow of the aforementioned spring. The trail takes you parallel to Jeremys Run, heading deeper into its valley. At 1.0 mile, meet the Knob Mountain Cutoff Trail, and begin the loop portion of the hike. ▶3 Here, turn right on the Knob Mountain Cutoff Trail. Immediately rock-hop Jeremys Run. Get water here since there is none for miles along Knob Mountain.

After crossing Jeremys Run, the trail switchbacks up a piney, rocky slope. The steep path makes use of a few old roads. Level off and come to the Knob Mountain Trail at 1.6 miles. ▶4 Turn

🍁 **Autumn Colors**

🔁 **Stream**

👣 **Steep**

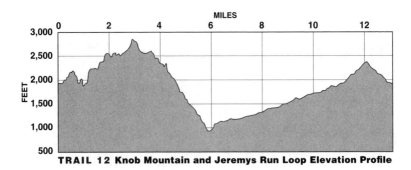

TRAIL 12 Knob Mountain and Jeremys Run Loop Elevation Profile

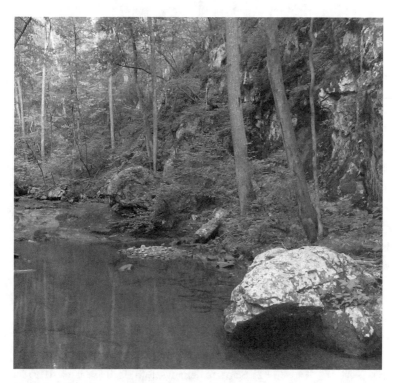

Jeremys Run *has clear, cool pools harboring brook trout.*

left, westerly, on the Knob Mountain Trail, following a former fire road. Here, the trail undulates over small prominences and outcrops, then dips to gaps, climbing ever so slightly toward the Knob Mountain summit. Views of the Shenandoah Valley are off to your right. The valley of Jeremys Run falls off to your left.

▲ Ridgeline

The trail is only partly canopied and often bordered with brush, including blackberries in summer. By mile 3.0, the ridge has become wide and level. This is grouse country; don't be surprised if a brown fowl flutters away at your feet. Just before reaching the summit, the former fire road ends at a concrete post. Continue forward on a footpath, making an abrupt ascent to the summit (2,865 feet) at 3.9 miles, which also has a concrete post. ▶5

The trail drops sharply off the summit. Look for the town of Luray and for Massanutten Mountain through the trees while working your way toward Jeremys Run. The path makes repeated switchbacks on the ridge. At 4.6 miles, the trail splits a gap and traces the left side of the ridge. Jeremys Run flows below you, and Neighbor Mountain rises across the valley. More switchbacks lead you through an area of pine trees and great views of the Shenandoah Valley. Pass a spring on your right at 6.0 miles. ▶6 It has been rocked in but may still need to be cleaned out.

Neighbor Mountain looms larger as you continue descending. Soon you can hear the intonations of Jeremys Run. At mile 6.7, pass a pioneer fence line and spring. Come to the creek crossing at the head of a nice pool, then intersect the Jeremys Run Trail at 7.1 miles. ▶7 Turn left and just ahead is the Neighbor Mountain Trail junction. Here are some good sitting rocks for a break.

Start up Jeremys Run Trail on a mild grade. Stone walls line the path. Regal white pines grow on former fields, but a few hemlocks are hanging on. Sycamores shade the stream, where brook trout gather in deep pools that double as places for sweaty hikers to cool off.

When rock bluffs crowd the stream, the trail crosses to the other side toward flatter terrain. Your next crossing is at 7.4 miles. This pattern continues time and again up the valley. These fords are dangerous only in times of high water. Most of the time you can make it dry-shod. The stream sometimes braids into dry channels. While walking up the valley, you are often 10 to 20 feet above the stream, allowing for good looks into the watercourse. Pass

Waterfall

a 10-foot, two-tier waterfall and popular swimming hole at 7.8 miles. ▶8

Swimming

Cross the run at 8.4 miles and then again at 9.2 and 9.5 miles. After 9.9 miles, the crossings become more frequent. A total of 16 crossings, including the first one at the lower end of the Knob Mountain Trail, brings you to the head of the valley and the junction with the Knob Mountain Cutoff Trail at mile 12.1. ▶9 Retrace your steps up the Jeremys Run Trail, coming once again to the AT. Head up the AT for 0.2 mile, then veer right up to the Elkwallow Picnic Ground, completing your loop at 13.1 miles. ▶10

MILESTONES

▶1	0.0	Elkwallow Picnic Ground at milepost 24.1
▶2	0.2	Pick up Jeremys Run Trail
▶3	1.0	Right on Knob Mountain Cutoff Trail
▶4	1.6	Left on Knob Mountain Trail
▶5	3.9	Knob Mountain summit
▶6	6.0	Spring to right of trail
▶7	7.1	Left on Jeremys Run Trail
▶8	7.8	Waterfall and swimming hole
▶9	12.1	Knob Mountain Cutoff Trail leaves left
▶10	13.1	Elkwallow Picnic Ground at milepost 24.1

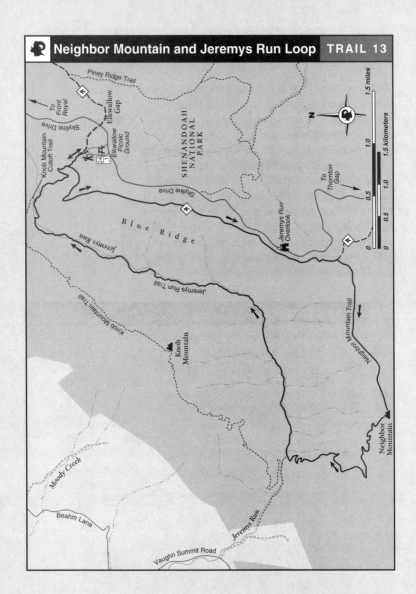

Neighbor Mountain and Jeremys Run Loop

In-shape hikers can complete this long loop in a day, but it makes an even better overnight backpack excursion. I have done it both ways. First, the circuit leaves Elkwallow Picnic Ground (which has water, restrooms, and shaded tables), then heads south-bound on the AT, traversing a pleasant stretch of the world's most famous pathway. Delve into solitude immediately upon joining the Neighbor Mountain Trail, and grab some views on your way to Jeremys Run, one of the prettiest and most productive trout streams in the park. Crisscross to the upper valley of Jeremys Run, then make a final climb, returning to the trailhead.

Best Time

From late spring through mid-fall, you can make the 15 crossings of Jeremys Run most safely and warmly. The stream will be lower then. Summer is great for fishing and swimming.

Finding the Trail

From Thornton Gap, take Skyline Drive north for 7.4 miles to Elkwallow Picnic Ground at milepost 24.1. Drive to the low end of the picnic area and park. The spur trail to the Appalachian Trail (AT) leaves here. The Elkwallow Wayside, a short dis-tance north on Skyline Drive, has a camp store and food offerings during the warm season if you don't feel like picnicking.

TRAIL USE
Dayhiking, Backpacking

LENGTH
14.0 miles,
8½–10 hours

**CUMULATIVE
ELEVATION +/-**
-1,650'/+1,650'

DIFFICULTY
– 1 2 3 4 **5** +

TRAIL TYPE
Loop

START & FINISH
N38° 45.715'
W78° 18.295'

FEATURES
Ridgeline
Stream
Summit
Autumn Colors
Waterfall
Wildflowers
Great Views
Steep
Secluded
Camping
Swimming

FACILITIES
Picnic area with water
    and restrooms
Camp store

Trail Description

Start your loop on the spur trail leaving Elkwallow Picnic Area to immediately intersect the AT. ►1 Veer left, heading downhill, southbound through woods. Pass a spur trail on your left to a cool spring just before meeting the Jeremys Run Trail at 0.2 mile. ►2 Make a left here, staying with the AT. Step over the outflow of the spring you just crossed. Begin a mile-long gentle ascent. At 0.7 mile the trail curves around a point and then enters laurel-oak woods atop the ridgeline. Views of Knob Mountain open to your right. Enjoy a forest cruise on a grass-lined, single-track ribbon in oak and hickory. The broken canopy presents obscured looks into the adjacent valleys and ridges. Begin a mild descent at 2.0 miles. At 2.4 miles, the Thornton River Trail leaves left. ►3 Continue the downgrade, cutting through brushy trees just below Jeremys Run Overlook at 3.1 miles. ►4 There is no trail access to the Skyline Drive viewpoint. Bottom out at 3.1 miles, then resume an uptick, meeting a spur trail left to Skyline Drive at 3.6 miles. ►5

Begin a winding climb up the western side of Neighbor Mountain, meeting the Neighbor Mountain Trail at 3.9 miles. ►6 Turn right, joining the well-maintained but faint-floored Neighbor

▲ Ridgeline

❦ Autumn Colors

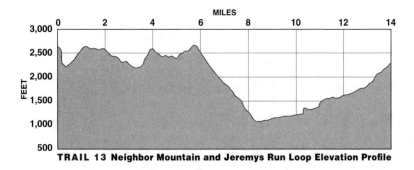

TRAIL 13 Neighbor Mountain and Jeremys Run Loop Elevation Profile

Mountain Trail. Expect solitude from here to Jeremys Run. The slender grassy ribbon meanders westerly beneath thick woodland that hosts a dense understory of mountain laurel and smaller trees. The woods become even more attractive and open with oaks and pine above and grass below. The ridgeline slopes sharply off both sides.

▲ Ridgeline

Hike over a knob to reach a conspicuous rock outcrop on your right at mile 4.9. Several dark rocks stand upright amid smaller rounded boulders. Hop up on a boulder and look over the Shenandoah Valley, which spreads to your right, and the mountains of the park's Central District, which hover on the skyline to your left. Someone must've imagined these upthrust rocks as militaries, for they are known as the "gendarmes," which are armed French police officers charged with maintaining order.

🏞 Great Views

Ahead, admire the manmade stonework on and astride the trail. Top out on Neighbor Mountain at 5.7 miles, marked with a concrete post. ▶7 The Potomac Appalachian Trail Club map states the viewless peak, cloaked in brushy, viney woods, to be 2,725 feet. Leave the mountain crest, northwest, descending the steep north slope of The Neighbor. You are in the process of dropping nearly 1,700 feet in 2.6 miles. Be glad you aren't going the other way!

🯄 Summit

🯄 Steep

The foot-pounding drop is moderated with switchbacks. Views between scraggly pines and low-growing blueberries open when the trail is on the ridge's south or west side. You are looking at the Three Sisters, a triple-knobbed ridge to the southwest, and the Shenandoah Valley beyond. The north side of Neighbor Mountain is more deeply wooded and sans vistas. At 7.4 miles, the trail dips to a hollow and briefly joins an old road beside a rocky streambed. ▶8 Reenter pine-oak woods, and resume switchbacking toward the valley floor. Eventually the rapids of Jeremys Run become audible, and

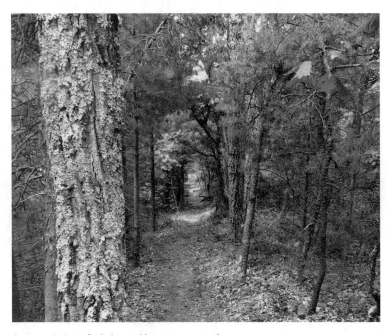

Oaks and pines *flank the Neighbor Mountain Trail.*

Stream

Waterfall

Swimming

the forest correspondingly thickens. Make the last switchback among lush, shaded ferns before meeting the Jeremys Run Trail at 8.3 miles. ▶9 If you want to explore a bit, walk left, downstream, down the Jeremy Run Trail. Some marvelous deep pools form below rock slab cascades. These swimming and fishing holes also sport big sunning rocks.

To continue on the loop hike, turn right onto Jeremys Run Trail. Make your first stream crossing, then come to a two-tier waterfall and swimming hole at 9.0 miles. ▶10 Rock walls line the path through here, and white pines rise over former trailside fields. Sycamores shade the stream where brook trout gather in deep pools. Where rock bluffs crowd Jeremys Run, the path crosses to the other side toward flatter terrain. This pattern of crowding and crossing continues up the valley. Most of the 15 crossings are in the upper valley. In times of high water these fords are dangerous, but most of the time you can cross the run dry-shod.

A steadier grade brings you to the upper valley and the junction with Knob Mountain Cutoff Trail at 13.0 miles. ►11 Stay right with the Jeremys Run Trail. Wind your way uphill to meet the AT at 13.8 miles. ►12 From here, backtrack to Elkwallow Picnic Ground, completing the hike at 14.0 miles. ►13

大	MILESTONES	
►1	0.0	Elkwallow Picnic Area at milepost 24.1
►2	0.2	Jeremys Run Trail leaves right
►3	2.4	Thornton River Trail leaves left
►4	3.1	Pass below Jeremys Run Overlook
►5	3.6	Spur to Skyline Drive
►6	3.9	Right on Neighbor Mountain Trail
►7	5.7	Neighbor Mountain summit
►8	7.4	Briefly join a roadbed along streambed
►9	8.3	Right on Jeremys Run Trail
►10	9.0	Waterfall and swimming hole on right
►11	13.0	Knob Mountain Cutoff Trail leaves left
►12	13.8	Rejoin the AT
►13	14.0	Elkwallow Picnic Ground

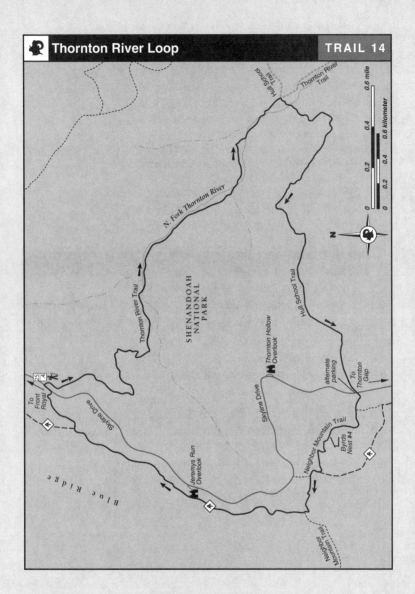

Thornton River Loop

TRAIL 14

0.6 mile
0.4
0.2
0
0.6 kilometer
0.4
0.2
0

N

Hull School Trail
Thornton River Trail

N. Fork Thornton River

Thornton River Trail

SHENANDOAH
NATIONAL
PARK

Hull School Trail

25
4

To
Front
Royal

Skyline Drive

Thornton Hollow Overlook

Skyline Drive

alternate parking

To
Thornton Gap

Jeremys Run Overlook

Neighbor Mountain Trail

Byrds
Nest #4

Blue Ridge

Neighbor
Mountain Trail

Thornton River Loop

This loop is a quiet hike through history, combined with a little high-country trekking. Leave Skyline Drive to walk the once settled Thornton Hollow. Here, relics of settlers are scattered onto the landscape. Walk along the alluring North Fork Thornton River, one of the park's more productive trout streams. Wander richly forested flats between creek crossings. Leave the lowlands on the Hull School Trail, angling up a once settled slope.

The path then crosses Skyline Drive and climbs a peak, where a day-use shelter stands. From here, descend to meet the Appalachian Trail (AT). Trace the AT northbound on a pleasant stretch of path back to the trailhead. I have backpacked this loop on a summer Saturday and not seen a soul. Mine was the only car in the lot too.

Best Time

Spring is a great time to view the wildflowers and see old homesites before the leaves grow back on the trees. Summer can be good for fishing and backpacking. The lesser-used loop offers decent solitude when other circuits may be busy. Late fall, when the leaves are off and the stream dead low, is also a good time.

Finding the Trail

Park in the area on the east side of Skyline Drive at milepost 25.4. The Thornton River Trail starts on the left side of the parking area.

TRAIL USE
Dayhiking, Backpacking
LENGTH
7.9 miles, 4½–5½ hours
CUMULATIVE ELEVATION +/-
-1,500'/+1,500'
DIFFICULTY
– 1 2 3 **4** 5 +
TRAIL TYPE
Loop
START & FINISH
N38° 43.435'
W78° 19.205'

FEATURES
Ridgeline
Summit
Stream
Autumn Colors
Wildflowers
Wildlife
Historic Interest
Secluded

FACILITIES
None

Trail Description

Start your hike by descending through a rocky oak-pine-maple-hickory forest on the Thornton Hollow Trail. ▶1 Trace an old settler roadbed on a blue-blazed track. Shortly step over a spring branch. It isn't long before you see the first rock pile, made by farmers clearing stony fields. Curve back north at 0.4 mile, still descending. White oaks and tulip trees are plentiful. The moderate slope made it easy for settlers to use this upper valley for pasture, even for growing corn.

At 0.9 mile, pass near an edifice-like rock pile. This square stone mound was added to year after year, in an attempt to clear what is now forested ground. Curve downhill to cross a tributary of the North Fork Thornton River at 1.0 mile. Rock walls line the settler road turned trail. But it wasn't just wagons and horses rumbling down this track—at 1.1 miles you can see the stripped remnants of an old jalopy. ▶2

Begin paralleling the branch, crossing it a second time. Sycamores, tulip trees, and other hardwoods rise over the waterway, along with white pines. Spicebush and stinging nettle share the understory. Come alongside the North Fork Thornton River. Flats widen on either side of the waterway.

Stream

Historic Interest

Autumn Colors

TRAIL 14 Thornton River Loop Elevation Profile

Continue down Thornton Hollow. At 1.9 miles, the river squeezes through a rock chute to your left in louder cascades and deeper pools. At 2.2 miles, a thickly wooded flat separates you from the river. Step over a stony tributary that may or may not be flowing. Cross the river at 2.3 miles. The North Fork Thornton River has a highly variable water flow, often braiding when high, but it should be fairly easy to cross except after storms. It is also one of Shenandoah's more productive brook trout streams.

 Wildflowers

At 2.6 miles, come alongside yet another rock wall. Pass over the outflow of the homesite spring. Just ahead, cross the river again. You are on the right-hand bank. Here, the valley widens. The imprint of humans is visible on both sides of the river. Look for roads, rock walls, and rusty artifacts. Remember, these are cultural resources of the park and should be left where they lay for others to enjoy. Keep down the hollow, and cross the river again at 2.8 miles. Enter a closing field to intersect the Hull School Trail at 2.9 miles. ▶3 The Hull School once stood to the right of you as you face downriver.

View relics of Shenandoah's pre-park residents on this hike.

Join the Hull School Trail, leading right to cross the watercourse at an island. Here, the trail jumps off and on old settler roads, evidenced by rutted beds and rock walls. Head uphill through straight-trunked cove hardwoods towering over a rock floor. Steepen at a pair of switchbacks, then step over a spring branch at 3.7 miles. This spring likely watered a homesite hereabouts. Continue up, heading off and on old roadbeds amid occasional flats. At 5.0 miles, the trail tops out. You are clearly on an old road, passing through farmland, despite being 2,300 feet in elevation and adjacent to the crest of the Blue Ridge.

Emerge onto Skyline Drive at 5.3 miles. ▶4 Here, the Rocky Branch Trail leaves left. This hike crosses Skyline Drive and heads up a gated fire road marking the beginning of the Neighbor Mountain Trail. Trace this double-track trail uphill past a clearing, then make a solid ascent to top out at Byrds Nest Shelter #4 at 5.6 miles. ▶5 This three-sided stone refuge looks east over a grassy clearing. Despite having a fireplace, it is for day use only.

Summit

From here, the yellow-blazed Neighbor Mountain Trail morphs into a single-track path. It drops westerly through pine-oak-laurel woods. Reach a trail junction at 6.0 miles. Here a spur trail leads right to the Neighbor Mountain parking area on Skyline Drive. Keep straight on the Neighbor Mountain Trail to meet the AT at 6.1 miles. ▶6 The hike turns right, northbound, on the heavily trod track. Soon pass another spur to Skyline Drive. Stay with the AT.

Ridgeline

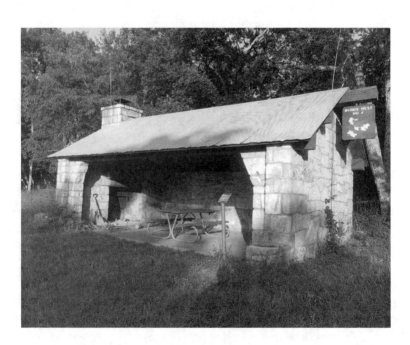

Byrds Nest Shelter #4, *atop a knob, proves an irresistible break spot.*

Bisect the brush below Jeremys Run Overlook at 6.9 miles. The AT makes for an easy, gently undulating walk under oaks. Meet the upper end of the Thornton River Trail at 7.6 miles. ►7 Turn right, dropping off the ridgeline. One final switchback drops you off just south of the Thornton River parking area, and you complete the loop hike at 7.9 miles. ►8

🍁 **Autumn Colors**

🚶 **MILESTONES**

►1	0.0	Thornton River parking area at milepost 25.4
►2	1.1	Old jalopy to the left of trail
►3	2.9	Right on Hull School Trail
►4	5.3	Cross Skyline Drive
►5	5.6	Byrds Nest Shelter #4
►6	6.1	Right on the AT
►7	7.6	Right on Thornton River Trail
►8	7.9	Thornton River parking area

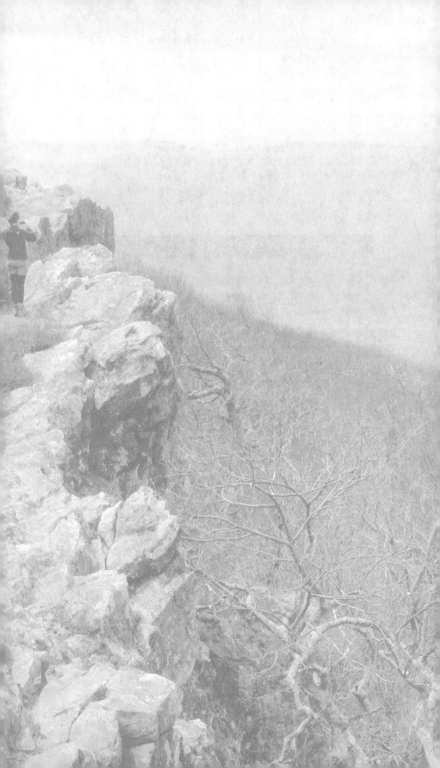

CHAPTER 2

Central District

15. Marys Rock via The Pinnacle
16. Hazel Falls and Cave
17. Hazel Country Loop
18. Corbin Cabin Hike
19. Old Rag Loop
20. Stony Man Loop
21. Robertson Mountain
22. Millers Head
23. Falls of Whiteoak Canyon
24. Cedar Run Falls
25. Hawksbill Summit
26. Rose River Falls Loop
27. Lewis Spring Falls Loop
28. Hazeltop and Rapidan Camp Loop
29. Bear Church Rock via Staunton River
30. Bear Church Rock from Bootens Gap
31. Conway River Loop
32. Pocosin Mission
33. South River Falls Loop
34. Saddleback Mountain Loop

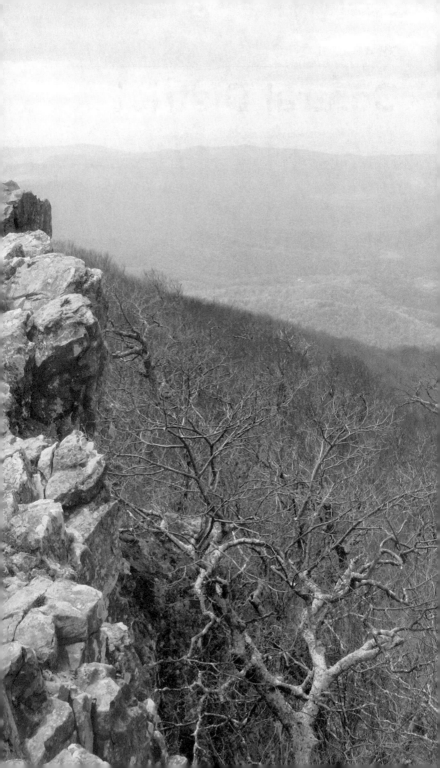

Central District

The Central District is the park's largest ranger district. Not surprisingly, it offers the most hiking opportunities, as well as other park possibilities, ranging from lodging to car camping to guided horseback riding and general visitor services. The Central District, quite wide in sections, begins at Thornton Gap in the north, with east-west US 211 bisecting the park while linking Sperryville and Luray. Skyline Drive runs for 34 miles through the district and accesses the area's major natural features, trailheads, campgrounds, and visitor facilities.

Heading south from Thornton Gap, you will first come to Hazel Country, a sizeable trail network that uses old pioneer paths and roads. Here, hikers will find pioneer evidence in the hills and hollows of the Hazel River and Hughes River Valleys. Loop hikes explore this land of the Old Dominion pioneer, as well as natural features such as Hazel Falls and Cave. Wonderful high-country hikes traverse the spine of the Blue Ridge, including the stellar view from Marys Rock, a must-visit destination. You will run into the first major visitor facility at Skyland, lodging quarters that predate the park's establishment. The shoulder of epic Stony Man Mountain, site of Skyland, is laced with exciting trails. Visit the open outcrops of Stony Man, or take a family hike to Millers Head, with its wide panoramas.

And then there's Old Rag. The deservedly popular peak is Virginia's contribution to great mountains of the world. The rock scramble up there is a thrilling challenge, and the views are simply spectacular. Robertson Mountain, Old Rag's neighbor, sports some fair vistas itself and is a destination solitude-seekers will better enjoy. Whiteoak Canyon is one of Shenandoah's most rugged gorges. Through it spills no less than seven major named waterfalls, along with innumerable lesser cataracts that together add up to one whitewater-filled valley. Whiteoak Canyon can be accessed from high and low. A parade of visitors reflects its convenient dual admission. The canyon of Cedar Run, just south of Whiteoak Canyon, is arguably even rougher. A stony-to-the-extreme trail leads hikers to more waterfalls and swimming holes. It's very popular too.

Overleaf and opposite: The sharp cliff *of Hawksbill (Trail 25) presents stellar vistas.*

Hawksbill, the park's highest peak at 4,050 feet, adds to the concentration of notable Central District hiking destinations. It's a fairly easy trek to this crested pinnacle, where a stony brow allows for sweeping views in all directions. Conveniently, an inlaid compass identifies adjacent mountains visible from the top of Hawksbill. Nearby, the Rose River Loop visits a pair of waterfalls and an old mine.

Big Meadows, a highland pasture, offers camping, a lodge, camp store, and visitor center where you can learn more about the park, purchase memorabilia, and participate in ranger programs. Stop by the visitor center when hiking to the vista at Blackrock Mountain and Lewis Falls, one of the park's highest elevation cataracts. Human history stands prominent again along Mill Prong, where President Herbert Hoover had his retreat, Rapidan Camp. You can tour this preserved aggregation of buildings along with natural features, such as Big Rock Falls and Hazeltop, one of the few areas in the park where rare spruce and fir trees cling to the heights.

More extensive treks incorporate state lands of the Rapidan Wildlife Management Area. Head up trout-rich Staunton River on your way to Bear Church Rock, a secluded vista with one of the greatest names in the entire Appalachian chain. Another hike heads deep down the Conway River Valley, a big and brawling stream. Your return trip takes you on the Bearfence Mountain Rock Scramble, a view-laden adventure through a boulder garden. Lewis Mountain, with its campground, cabins, and fine picnic area, offers a tamer experience.

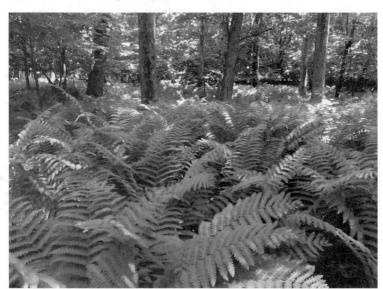

Ferns *at Stony Man Loop (Trail 20)*

Things quiet down near Pocosin Mission, a short walk from Skyline Drive. Visit the ruins of a Christian ministry from pre-park days. Hikers often incorporate a meal into their hike at rustic South River Picnic Area. One walk leads to South River Falls, a cataract you can enjoy from above and below. Wildflowers carpet this valley in spring. Hikers seeking solitude make a loop over Saddleback Mountain, contemplating nature on nature's terms. US 33, which connects Elkton in the west to Stanardsville in the east, marks the southern boundary of the Central District.

Permits

Permits are not required for dayhiking. Backpackers must get a backcountry permit to stay in the backcountry. Simple self-registration stations are located at Thornton Gap Entrance Station, Big Meadows Visitor Center, and Swift Run Gap Entrance Station on Skyline Drive and at Old Rag Fee Station on the park's east side.

Maps

For the Central District, here are the USGS 7.5-minute (1:24,000-scale) topographic quadrangles that you will need, listed in the order that you will need them as you hike along your route.

Trail 15: *Old Rag Mountain* and *Thornton Gap*
Trail 16: *Thornton Gap*
Trail 17: *Thornton Gap* and *Old Rag Mountain*
Trail 18: *Old Rag Mountain*
Trail 19: *Old Rag Mountain*
Trail 20: *Big Meadows* and *Old Rag Mountain*
Trail 21: *Big Meadows* and *Old Rag Mountain*
Trail 22: *Big Meadows*
Trail 23: *Old Rag Mountain*
Trail 24: *Big Meadows* and *Old Rag Mountain*
Trail 25: *Big Meadows*
Trail 26: *Big Meadows*
Trail 27: *Big Meadows*
Trail 28: *Big Meadows* and *Fletcher*
Trail 29: *Madison* and *Fletcher*
Trail 30: *Fletcher*
Trail 31: *Fletcher*
Trail 32: *Fletcher*
Trail 33: *Elkton East* and *Fletcher*
Trail 34: *Elkton East* and *Swift Run Gap*

Central District

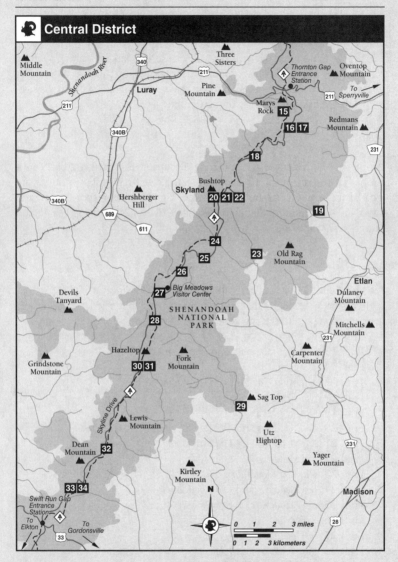

TRAIL FEATURES TABLE

Central District

TRAIL	Difficulty	Length	Type	USES & ACCESS	TERRAIN	NATURE	OTHER
15	3	7.2	Out & Back	Dayhiking	Ridgeline	Autumn Colors	Great Views, Geologic Interest
16	3	5.2	Out & Back	Dayhiking, Child-Friendly	Ridgeline, Stream, Waterfall	Autumn Colors, Wildflowers	Geologic Interest
17	4	7.9	Loop	Dayhiking, Backpacking	Ridgeline, Stream	Autumn Colors, Wildflowers	Historic Interest, Secluded
18	3	2.8	Out & Back	Dayhiking	Ridgeline, Stream	Autumn Colors, Wildflowers	Historic Interest
19	5	9.1	Loop	Dayhiking, Pets Prohibited	Summit, Ridgeline, Stream	Autumn Colors, Wildflowers	Great Views, Geologic Interest
20	3	3.4	Loop	Dayhiking, Pets Prohibited	Summit, Ridgeline	Autumn Colors	Great Views, Geologic Interest, Historic Interest
21	4	6.8	Out & Back	Dayhiking	Summit, Ridgeline, Stream	Autumn Colors	Great Views
22	2	1.4	Out & Back	Dayhiking, Child-Friendly	Ridgeline	Autumn Colors	Great Views
23	4	5.2	Out & Back	Dayhiking	Stream, Waterfall	Wildflowers	Great Views, Geologic Interest, Steep
24	4	3.4	Out & Back	Dayhiking	Stream, Waterfall	Autumn Colors, Wildflowers	Geologic Interest, Steep
25	2	2.2	Out & Back	Dayhiking	Summit	Autumn Colors	Great Views
26	3	4.0	Loop	Dayhiking, Backpacking	Stream, Waterfall	Autumn Colors, Wildflowers	Geologic Interest, Historic Interest
27	3	3.3	Loop	Dayhiking	Summit, Ridgeline, Stream, Waterfall	Autumn Colors, Wildflowers	Great Views, Geologic Interest
28	4	7.2	Loop	Dayhiking, Backpacking	Summit, Ridgeline, Stream, Waterfall	Autumn Colors, Wildflowers, Wildlife	Great Views, Historic Interest
29	5	7.6	Out & Back	Dayhiking, Backpacking	Ridgeline, Stream, Waterfall	Autumn Colors	Great Views, Geologic Interest, Swimming, Secluded
30	4	9.4	Out & Back	Dayhiking	Ridgeline	Autumn Colors	Great Views, Geologic Interest, Secluded
31	5	12.0	Loop	Dayhiking, Backpacking, Pets Prohibited	Ridgeline, Stream, Waterfall	Autumn Colors, Wildflowers, Old-Growth	Great Views, Geologic Interest, Historic Interest
32	2	2.0	Out & Back	Dayhiking, Child-Friendly	Ridgeline	Autumn Colors, Wildflowers, Old-Growth	Great Views, Historic Interest
33	3	4.5	Loop	Dayhiking	Stream, Waterfall	Autumn Colors, Wildflowers	Geologic Interest
34	2	3.9	Loop	Dayhiking, Child-Friendly	Ridgeline	Autumn Colors, Wildflowers	Secluded

Legend

USES & ACCESS
- Dayhiking
- Backpacking
- Child-Friendly
- Pets Prohibited

TYPE
- Loop
- Out & Back
- DIFFICULTY - 1 2 3 4 5 + (less ... more)

TERRAIN
- Summit
- Ridgeline
- Stream
- Waterfall

NATURE
- Autumn Colors
- Wildflowers
- Wildlife
- Old-Growth

FEATURES
- Great Views
- Geologic Interest
- Historic Interest
- Swimming
- Secluded
- Steep

Central District

TRAIL 15

Dayhiking

7.2 miles, Out & Back

Difficulty: 1 2 **3** 4 5

Marys Rock via The Pinnacle 121

The hike over The Pinnacle to Marys Rock traverses the most spectacular section of the Appalachian Trail in the park. Views are expansive and frequent after leaving the Pinnacles picnic area. A climb leads to The Pinnacle with an outstanding vista. Finally reach what Shenandoah old-timers believe to be the best vista in the entire park—Marys Rock.

TRAIL 16

Dayhiking,

Child-Friendly

5.2 miles, Out & Back

Difficulty: 1 2 **3** 4 5

Hazel Falls and Cave 127

This hike takes you into "Hazel Country," a heavily settled area in pre-park days. The route traverses hill and hollow for the Hazel River, where a rock indentation forms a natural shelter beside a waterfall, all within a deep stone cathedral.

TRAIL 17

Dayhiking, Backpacking

7.9 miles, Loop

Difficulty: 1 2 3 **4** 5

Hazel Country Loop 131

This circuit heads down to the Hazel River, traveling over a series of old mountain roads turned trails and visiting a series of flat-topped mountains, stomping grounds of pre-park settlers, where fields, schools, and farms once stood. Elevation changes on this solitude-laden hike are neither steep nor severe, making it a favorable walk for pioneer history buffs.

Corbin Cabin Hike 135

TRAIL 18

Visit an intact, authentic Shenandoah pioneer cabin, via a steep trail created by settlers. Corbin Cabin, set in the upper Hughes River, is a naturally alluring locale. The cabin, available for overnight rental, requires a 1,000-foot descent and ascent.

Dayhiking
2.8 miles, Out & Back
Difficulty: 1 2 **3** 4 5

Old Rag Loop 139

TRAIL 19

This well-loved Shenandoah classic is the most difficult hike in this entire guidebook. Strike up the north slope of Old Rag, emerging onto a massive granite slab, revealing incredible panoramas. Enter a maze of boulders, with some bona fide rock scrambling to reach the summit with stellar views. Leave the rugged mountaintop, and reenter the lowlands via the pretty valley of Brokenback Run on a foot-relieving gravel fire road.

Dayhiking,
Pets Prohibited
9.1 miles, Loop
Difficulty: 1 2 3 4 **5**

Stony Man Loop 145

TRAIL 20

Hike to the summit of Stony Man Mountain, where cliffs rise 3,000 feet above the Shenandoah Valley and present superlative panoramas. Take the Little Stony Man Trail to Little Stony Man, where more overlooks await. Return along the Passamaquoddy Trail, where still more views can be seen. Stop by Furnace Spring, once used in a copper mining operation, before completing this highlight-laden loop.

Dayhiking,
Pets Prohibited
3.4 miles, Loop
Difficulty: 1 2 **3** 4 5

Robertson Mountain 151

TRAIL 21

Before reaching this lesser-visited peak, explore a highland cove and wetland on the all-access Limberlost Trail. Join Old Rag Fire Road, where the walking is easy. A more traditional single-track foot trail takes you the last mile to the outcrops of Robertson Mountain. At the summit, various rocky points avail sweeping views in three directions.

Dayhiking
6.8 miles, Out & Back
Difficulty: 1 2 3 **4** 5

TRAIL 22

Dayhiking,
Child-Friendly
1.4 miles, Out & Back
Difficulty: 1 **2** 3 4 5

Millers Head 157
Start high, adjacent to Skyland Resort facilities, and surmount a wooded knob to enjoy the view from Bushy Head. From there, you wind westerly, passing a wonderful unnamed view from an outcrop. At the trail's end, a stone platform allows widespread westerly panoramas from the bottom of Shenandoah Valley to West Virginia and points between.

TRAIL 23

Dayhiking
5.2 miles, Out & Back
Difficulty: 1 2 3 **4** 5

Falls of Whiteoak Canyon 163
Explore six sequentially numbered falls while ascending a rugged gorge with everywhere-you-look beauty. Top out on a rock promontory with a view of the uppermost falls. Beware the crowds during nice weather.

TRAIL 24

Dayhiking
3.4 miles, Out & Back
Difficulty: 1 2 3 **4** 5

Cedar Run Falls 169
This hike leads into rugged upper Cedar Run Canyon. The steep trail passes countless cascades spilling down the narrow, boulder-laden gorge. The trip to the falls is slow because you need to watch your footing and stop often to admire the scenery.

TRAIL 25

Dayhiking
2.2 miles, Out & Back
Difficulty: 1 **2** 3 4 5

Hawksbill Summit 175
This easy, favorite hike starts at a high elevation and gets to the top of things in Shenandoah. Along the way you enter a "sky island" of Canadian-type forest. Outcrops below the summit are just warm-ups for the nearly 360-degree view from the summit of Hawksbill.

Rose River Falls Loop 179

This loop hike is long on beauty but sometimes short on solitude. First, visit Dark Hollow Falls. Next, hike downstream along Hogcamp Branch, passing numerous cascades along arguably the prettiest stream in the park. Bridge Hogcamp Branch, then view remnants of an old copper mine. Ascend to Rose River Falls before returning to the trailhead.

TRAIL 26

Dayhiking, Backpacking
4.0 miles, Loop
Difficulty: 1 2 **3** 4 5

Lewis Spring Falls Loop 185

This popular, high-country loop near Big Meadows heads northbound on the Appalachian Trail, climbing to Blackrock and its stellar views. From there, the hike passes more interesting rock features and then joins the Lewis Falls Trail, leading to a loud and dramatic cataract.

TRAIL 27

Dayhiking
3.3 miles, Loop
Difficulty: 1 2 **3** 4 5

Hazeltop and Rapidan Camp Loop.. 191

This loop leads over Hazeltop, third highest peak in the park, and then traces attractive Laurel Prong Trail down to Rapidan Camp, President Herbert Hoover's woodland getaway. There's much to see at the camp; you can even embark on a self-guided interpretive tour. Return to Milam Gap via Mill Prong Trail, and view Big Rock Falls along the way.

TRAIL 28

Dayhiking, Backpacking
7.2 miles, Loop
Difficulty: 1 2 3 **4** 5

Bear Church Rock via
Staunton River 197

Hike up the Staunton River Valley, a classic mountain vale centered with a pool-and-chute trout stream. Wind into the high-country, and emerge at a rock promontory that offers both solitude and first-rate views.

TRAIL 29

Dayhiking, Backpacking
7.6 miles, Out & Back
Difficulty: 1 2 3 4 **5**

TRAIL 30

Dayhiking
9.4 miles, Out & Back
Difficulty: 1 2 3 **4** 5

Bear Church Rock from Bootens Gap 201
This solitude-laden high-country hike leads along the ridge of Jones Mountain to a fine view. The hiking along Jones Mountain is some of Shenandoah's finest. Stay above 3,000 feet on trail that is never steep for long and mostly level, making it a glorious 9 mountain miles.

TRAIL 31

Dayhiking, Backpacking,
Pets Prohibited
12.0 miles, Loop
Difficulty: 1 2 3 4 **5**

Conway River Loop 205
Leave the Blue Ridge, and follow the scenic Conway River through an archetypal Appalachian valley. Next, head into the high country on the seldom trampled Slaughter Trail, passing pioneer homesites. Complete your trip by clambering over Bearfence Mountain, with its 360-degree views, on a short but challenging rock scramble.

TRAIL 32

Dayhiking,
Child-Friendly
2.0 miles, Out & Back
Difficulty: 1 **2** 3 4 5

Pocosin Mission 213
Take a short walk into the past. The wide and easy Pocosin Fire Road heads to ruins of the Pocosin Mission. Explore the ruins of the mission and other nearby signs of habitation on a child-friendly trek.

TRAIL 33

Dayhiking
4.5 miles, Loop
Difficulty: 1 2 **3** 4 5

South River Falls Loop 219
Make an easy descent to see South River Falls drop 80 feet over a rock face from a perched vista. Go farther to the base of the falls in a rich spring wildflower zone. Climb from the South River watershed back to the former mountaintop pastureland. The falls are worth the exercise.

Saddleback Mountain Loop 225

This loop allows you to enjoy a relatively level, easy stretch of the world's most famous footpath and then circle back on a seldom-used, solitude-soaked side trail. The elevation changes along this hike are not great, making it accessible for less able hikers or those with young families ready to try a longer hike.

TRAIL 34

Dayhiking,
Child-Friendly
3.9 miles, Loop
Difficulty: 1 **2** 3 4 5

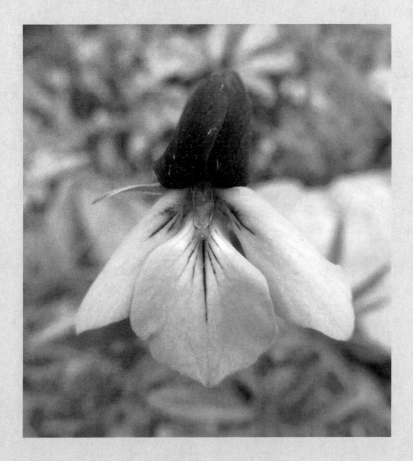

Delicate violet *graces the forest floor near Lewis Spring Falls (Trail 27).*

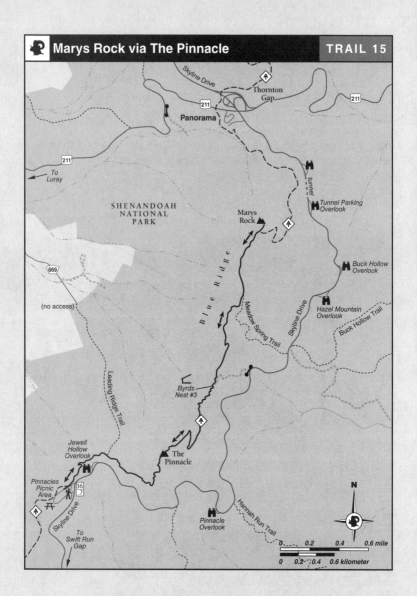

SHENANDOAH
NATIONAL
PARK

Skyline Drive

Thornton
Gap

211

211

Panorama

211

To
Luray

669

(no access)

tunnel

Tunnel Parking
Overlook

Marys
Rock

Buck Hollow
Overlook

Blue Ridge

Meadow Spring Trail

Hazel Mountain
Overlook

Buck Hollow Trail

Leading Ridge Trail

Skyline Drive

Byrds
Nest #3

Jewell
Hollow
Overlook

The Pinnacle

Pinnacles
Picnic
Area

36
.7

Skyline Drive

To
Swift Run
Gap

Hannah Run Trail

Pinnacle
Overlook

N

0   0.2   0.4   0.6 mile

0   0.2   0.4   0.6 kilometer

Marys Rock via The Pinnacle

The hike over The Pinnacle to Marys Rock traverses the most spectacular section of the AT through Shenandoah National Park. The views are expansive and frequent. And hiking to a view is always more rewarding than driving to a view. Panoramas open up shortly after you leave Pinnacles Picnic Area. A climb leads you to The Pinnacle, which has an outstanding vista. Still more views await before what many Shenandoah old-timers feel is the best vista in the entire park—Marys Rock. This hike's rewards far outstrip the effort it requires. Its elevation changes only amount to climbs and drops of 450 feet each—not bad for this park, not bad at all.

Best Time

Fall through spring is the best period for maximizing the multiple stunning views along this ridgeline. The weather is mild even in summer, since the trail never dips below 3,200 feet.

Finding the Trail

The Pinnacles Picnic Area is located at milepost 36.7 on Skyline Drive. From the Thornton Gap Entrance Station, take Skyline Drive south for 5.2 miles to the Pinnacles Picnic Area entrance. Pick up the Appalachian Trail (AT) on your right as you top out in the picnic area, before the road starts looping around. If the picnic area is closed (as it is in winter), simply start at Jewell Hollow Overlook at milepost 36.4. Pick up the AT at the south end of the overlook.

TRAIL USE
Dayhiking

LENGTH
7.2 miles, 4–5 hours

CUMULATIVE ELEVATION +/-
+450'/-450'

DIFFICULTY
– 1 2 **3** 4 5 +

TRAIL TYPE
Out & Back

START & FINISH
N38° 37.483'
W78° 20.539'

FEATURES
Ridgeline
Autumn Colors
Geologic Interest
Great Views

FACILITIES
Picnic tables
Water
Restrooms

Trail Description

Pick up the AT in the grassy margin to the right of the picnic area entrance road. ▶1 Head right, northbound, for Jewell Hollow Overlook. Pass some spruce trees that were probably planted. Views immediately open to your left as you travel along a stony upthrust escarpment. Dip to reach the Jewell Hollow Overlook at 0.2 mile. ▶2 The AT goes south a short distance before making a switchback to head north. Come to a small field below the overlook. Enjoy an unobstructed opening to the west. Lake Arrowhead lies below. Begin to climb beyond the field. Reenter woodland, coming to a trail junction at 0.5 mile. ▶3 Pass the Leading Ridge Trail, and continue north on the AT.

The path tunnels through an understory of mountain laurel in dense woodland. At 0.9 mile enter a forest area littered with massive gray boulders. The trees are short because of thin soils and rough climatic conditions atop the mountains. Meander amid the boulders, watching for unusual stacked stones that seem likely to fall. Open onto The Pinnacle (3,730 feet) at mile 1.2. ▶4 The rock outcrop has a sheer drop-off. Be prepared for an incredible view of Virginia mountains and valleys to the west. You can see Luray below and on a clear day look north at the balance of the park, including

> From this trail, soak in what is arguably the best panorama in the park.

 Autumn Colors

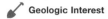 Geologic Interest

TRAIL 15 Marys Rock via The Pinnacle Elevation Profile

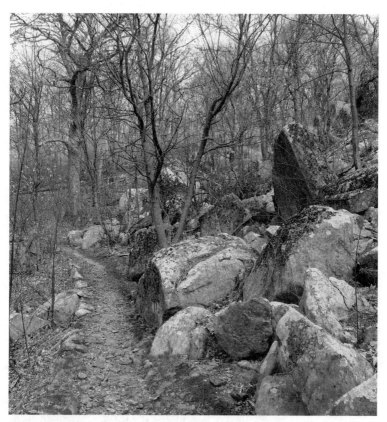

Massive gray boulders *border the cleared track of the Appalachian Trail.*

your destination—Marys Rock, a mere bump along the ridge from here. Be careful on these jagged, uneven rocks.

 Great Views

The AT continues north and descends a series of switchbacks in very stony woods. Slip over to the southeast side of the mountain. In a gap, reach the Byrds Nest Shelter #3 at 2.1 miles. ▶5 The three-sided camping structure is open to AT thru-hikers, defined as three consecutive nights or longer on the AT. This stone shelter has a picnic table and provides a respite from the elements, but don't expect the water fountain to work. A privy stands just ahead. Follow the service road that leads from the shelter to Skyline Drive for a short distance. Veer left at the intersection, staying on the AT. The service road drops right to a spring.

Another westward view opens at mile 2.5, soon after a switchback to the left. You can also look back at The Pinnacle and its outcrops. A grassy flat here beckons a rest. Ahead, a rock promontory offers more looks at 2.7 miles, including Stony Man Mountain. The Meadow Spring Trail leaves right at mile 2.9. ▶6 Begin climbing for a quarter mile. The trail levels as it approaches the backside of Marys Rock. Continue downhill to the Marys Rock spur trail at 3.5 miles. ▶7 Turn left on the spur trail and rise to Marys Rock, reaching it at 3.6 miles. ▶8

Great Views

The panorama from the huge outcrop ranges far and wide. Choose your viewing spot. To the north easy views of many Blue Ridge peaks open. The town of Luray and the Shenandoah Valley are visible to the west. The Thornton Gap Entrance Station stands clearly below. Agile hikers can walk to the highest rock of the outcrop, due south from the main overlook. The top is marked with a pair of USGS survey markers. From there, you can see in every direction. Decide for yourself if Marys Rock has the best view in the park. Just be careful doing it. It is undeniably one of the best and a personal favorite.

Great Views

🚶 MILESTONES

►1	0.0	Pinnacles Picnic Area
►2	0.2	Jewell Hollow Overlook
►3	0.5	Leading Ridge Trail leads left
►4	1.2	Vista from The Pinnacle
►5	2.1	Byrds Nest Shelter #3
►6	2.9	Meadow Spring Trail leaves right
►7	3.5	Spur trail to Marys Rock
►8	3.6	Marys Rock

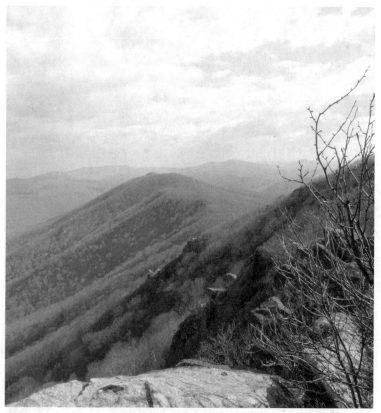

The Pinnacle *offers northward views of the Blue Ridge and the north district of the park beyond.*

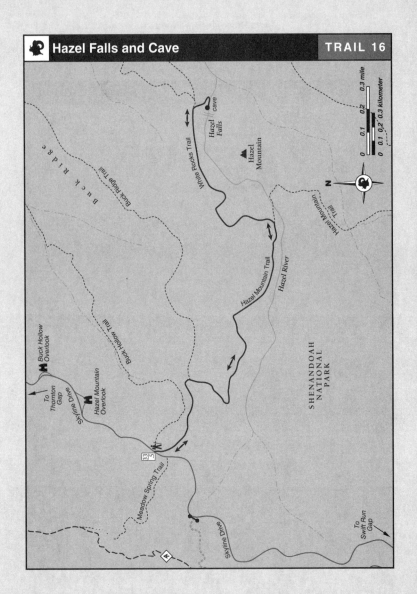

Hazel Falls and Cave

This hike takes you into "Hazel Country," a heavily settled area in pre-park days. The route traverses hill and hollow for the Hazel River, where a rock indentation forms a natural shelter beside a waterfall, all within a deep stone cathedral. All in all, it's a good destination. The difficulty of this hike is hard to rate: The first 2.4-mile portion is a moderate stroll on old settler roads, but the last 0.3-mile trek to the cave and falls is on a steep, rough footpath. Though rugged, this section is short; all but small children should make it.

Best Time

The falls flow more during winter and spring. On summer weekends fellow hikers head to the glen where the falls and cave are enclosed. Winter offers solitude aplenty and an iced-over cataract.

Finding the Trail

The trailhead is located east of milepost 33.5 of Skyline Drive at Meadow Spring. The parking area is on the east side of Skyline Drive. It is 2 miles south of the Thornton Gap Entrance Station on Skyline Drive.

Trail Description

Leave Skyline Drive on the Hazel Mountain Trail, formerly the Hazel Mountain Fire Road. ▶1 Come to a trail junction at 0.4 mile. ▶2 Veer right, still

TRAIL USE
Dayhiking,
Child-Friendly

LENGTH
5.2 miles, 2½–3½ hours

**CUMULATIVE
ELEVATION +/-**
-950'/+950'

DIFFICULTY
– 1 2 **3** 4 5 +

TRAIL TYPE
Out & Back

START & FINISH
N38° 38.298'
W78° 18.828'

FEATURES
Stream
Ridgeline
Waterfall
Autumn Colors
Geologic Interest
Wildflowers

FACILITIES
None

▲ Ridgeline

on the Hazel Mountain Trail, as the Buck Ridge Trail drops left. Striped maples crowd the path and form a dense canopy overhead. Striped maples are a smaller tree, easily recognized by the vertical stripes on green bark and typical maple leaves, albeit larger than red maples. It grows primarily throughout the northeast, where it is nicknamed "moosewood." Striped maples stretch south along the spine of the Appalachians down to Georgia. "Moosewood" derives from moose feeding on its bark in winter. Deer, beavers, and rabbits also feed on striped maples during the cold season.

Soon the trail bears left, levels out, and crosses several small spring branches dribbling down Buck Ridge. In some places, the forest is nearly devoid of ground cover, revealing the spindly trunks of second-growth even-aged trees, an aftereffect of the wildfires in 2000.

The trail sidles alongside the Hazel River at mile 1.0. The valley spreads wide into a cove—farmland way back when. Continue along the river, and turn left on the White Rocks Trail at mile 1.6. ▶3 The path ascends slightly, leaving Hazel River, then levels out along an old road shaded by tulips and maples. Other old roads veer off this trail, but the main path is evident. Large boulders are strewn about the forest, which morphs to pine and chestnut

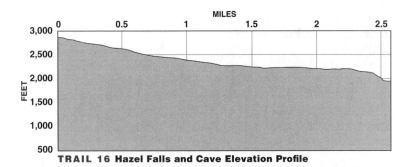

TRAIL 16 Hazel Falls and Cave Elevation Profile

oak as the trail tops out on the ridge. Wild azaleas bloom in May.

 Wildflowers

The trail becomes rockier and descends somewhat. A watery symphony drifts from below. Come to a trail junction at mile 2.4. ▶4 The White Rocks Trail continues forward, while the now-designated Cave and Falls Trail footpath veers right. Follow the Cave and Falls Trail downhill. Immediately pass a "No Camping" sign. The trail then dives down a steep path mitigated by stone steps. Carefully descend to the river. Hazel Mountain rises across the way. River cascades spill down the valley below.

Stream

Reach the river at 2.5 miles. Notice the peeling trunks of the many yellow birches. Turn right, following the footpath upstream. Pass a sizeable trailside tulip tree as you dance betwixt boulders. Reach the rock shelter on your right just before the waterfall. A natural rock amphitheater enfolds the scene. The rock indentation lies on your right at the base of a huge, granite bluff—quite a sturdy roof. ▶5 The cave is about 10 feet deep, 25 feet wide, and 7 feet high. It gets a little deeper in one spot. Hazel Falls slices about 25 feet down a narrow chute into a deep pool, and is but one piece of this picturesque mountain mosaic.

Geologic Interest

Waterfall

The rock notch makes this a good rainy-day destination. If you explore the rest of the boulders carefully, you will find more open overhangs, as well as other waterfall observation points. Relax and take it all in.

⚐	MILESTONES	
▶1	0.0	Meadow Spring parking area at milepost 33.5
▶2	0.4	Stay right as Buck Ridge Trail leaves left
▶3	1.6	Left on White Rocks Trail
▶4	2.4	Right on Cave and Falls Trail
▶5	2.6	Hazel Falls and Cave

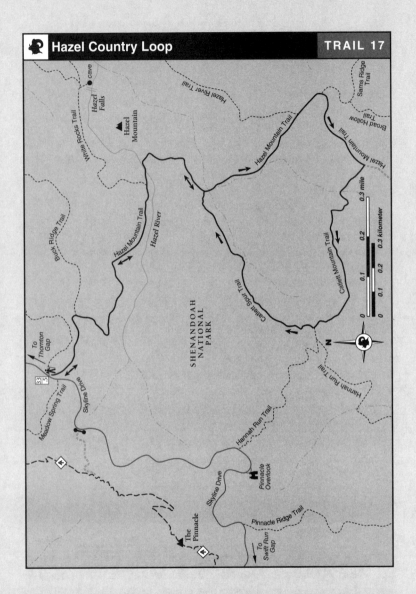

Sams Ridge Trail

Broad Hollow Trail

Hazel River Trail

White Rocks Trail

cave

Hazel Falls

Hazel Mountain

Hazel Mountain Trail

Hazel Mountain Trail

Buck Ridge Trail

Hazel Mountain Trail

Hazel River

Catlett Mountain Trail

Catlett Spur Trail

SHENANDOAH
NATIONAL
PARK

0.3 mile

0.3 kilometer

0.2

0.2

0.1

0.1

0

0

To
Thornton
Gap

33
5

Hannah Run Trail

Meadow Spring Trail

Skyline Drive

Hannah Run Trail

N

Skyline Drive

Pinnacle
Overlook

The Pinnacle

Pinnacle Ridge Trail

To
Swift Run
Gap

Hazel Country Loop

This circuit meanders through "Hazel Country," one of the most heavily settled areas before the park was established. Head down to the Hazel River, then travel over a series of old mountain roads turned trails, and visit a series of flat-topped mountains, stomping grounds of pre-park settlers, where fields, schools, and farms once stood. Though it won't jump out at you, pre-park history is all over this loop. Hikers can look for stone fences, rock piles, forgotten traces, flats where buildings once stood, and more. Leave your discoveries for others to enjoy. The elevation changes on this solitude-laden hike are neither steep nor severe, making it a favorable walk for pioneer history buffs who want a relaxing amble in national park–worthy scenery. Backpackers have their choice of level campsites.

Best Time

Pre-park pioneer homesites show up clearer when the trees don't have leaves. Spring has wildflowers, and the varied forest is a cornucopia of color in fall. Hikers can find solitude almost anytime, especially on the loop portion of the hike.

Finding the Trail

The trailhead is east of milepost 33.5 of Skyline Drive at Meadow Spring. The parking area is on the east side of Skyline Drive. It is 2 miles south of the Thornton Gap Entrance Station on Skyline Drive.

TRAIL USE
Dayhiking, Backpacking

LENGTH
7.9 miles, 4–5½ hours

CUMULATIVE ELEVATION +/-
-1,200'/+1,200'

DIFFICULTY
– 1 2 3 **4** 5 +

TRAIL TYPE
Loop

START & FINISH
N38° 38.298'
W78° 18.828'

FEATURES
Ridgeline
Stream
Autumn Colors
Wildflowers
Historic Interest
Secluded

FACILITIES
None

Trail Description

▲ **Ridgeline**

✹ **Autumn Colors**

▶ **Stream**

▶ **Stream**

Pick up the Hazel Mountain Trail, ▶1 leaving Skyline Drive on a gentle downgrade, immediately passing the Buck Hollow Trail. Come to a trail junction at 0.4 mile. ▶2 Veer right, still on the Hazel Mountain Trail, as the Buck Ridge Trail drops left. The path turns left and levels out. Step over several small spring branches dribbling down Buck Ridge. At 1.0 mile, the sounds of smallish Hazel River drift up to the trail. White pines shade the widening valley, lands that were plowed a century back. Continue downriver, meeting the White Rocks Trail at 1.6 miles. ▶3 Stay straight with the Hazel Mountain Trail, leaving other hikers who are mostly heading for Hazel Falls and Cave behind. Dip to rock-hop the Hazel River. The hike gently surmounts a low hill dividing Hazel River from Runyon Run.

Come to another trail junction beside Runyon Run at 2.2 miles. ▶4 Turn left here, still on the Hazel Mountain Trail to rock-hop wide and shallow Runyon Run. The wide path gently ascends a broad wooded valley. Its cultivation potential is evident to hikers today as it was to settlers way back when. At 2.8 miles, the Hazel River Trail leaves left, but this hike continues to follow the Hazel Mountain Trail in its meanderings. ▶5 This flat-for-mountain land

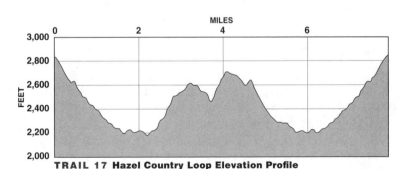

TRAIL 17 Hazel Country Loop Elevation Profile

reveals rock walls and other settler evidence. The 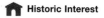 **Historic Interest**
old Hazel School was located hereabouts.

Stay with the Hazel Mountain Trail at 3.0 miles
as the Sams Ridge Trail leaves left. ▶6 All these trails
were once settlement roads traveled by mountaineers,
now reverted to scenic mountain paths reverberating
nothing but solitude. At 3.5 miles, in yet another
flat, turn right on the Catlett Mountain Trail. ▶7 The ▲ **Ridgeline**
path drops to a laurel-filled streamlet and then climbs
through a spindly woodland covering former fields.

Top out at 4.1 miles, and drop to a gap. Look for
an odd trailside sinkhole before coming to another
intersection at 4.7 miles. ▶8 This circuit turns
right onto the Catlett Spur Trail. Follow a shallow
wooded valley downhill, crossing the upper reaches
of Runyon Run on a rocky pioneer road. Crisscross
the gurgling stream that runs through the center of
the mountain flat. The old road curves away from the  **Stream**
valley center. Big stone walls line the woods here.

Return to the Hazel Mountain Trail at 5.7 miles,
completing the loop portion of the hike. ▶9 It is now **Discover**
a 2.2-mile backtrack to the trailhead. ▶10 Take your **Shenandoah's**
time, and look for more signs of pioneers on your **pioneer past.**
return route.

🚶	**MILESTONES**	
▶1	0.0	Meadow Spring parking area at milepost 33.5
▶2	0.4	Buck Ridge Trail leaves left
▶3	1.6	Cross Hazel River
▶4	2.2	Cross Runyon Run
▶5	2.8	Hazel River Trail leaves left
▶6	3.0	Sams Ridge Trail leaves left
▶7	3.5	Join Catlett Mountain Trail
▶8	4.7	Join Catlett Spur Trail
▶9	5.7	Rejoin Hazel Mountain Trail and backtrack
▶10	7.9	Meadow Spring parking area at milepost 33.5

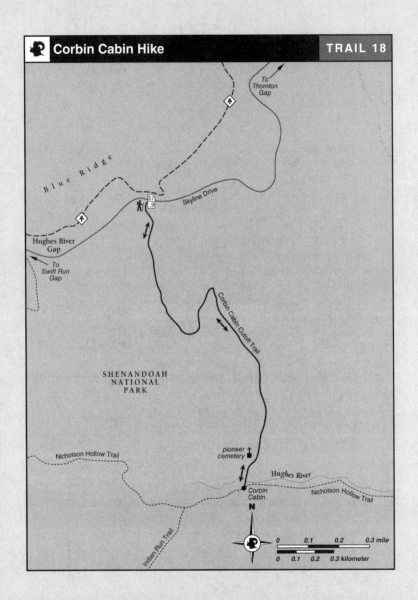

To
Thornton
Gap

Blue Ridge

Skyline Drive

37
9

Hughes River
Gap

To
Swift Run
Gap

Corbin Cabin Cutoff Trail

SHENANDOAH
NATIONAL
PARK

Nicholson Hollow Trail

pioneer
cemetery

Hughes River

Corbin
Cabin

Nicholson Hollow Trail

Indian Run Trail

N

| 0 | 0.1 | 0.2 | 0.3 mile |

| 0 | 0.1 | 0.2 | 0.3 kilometer |

Corbin Cabin Hike

Do you want to visit an intact, authentic Shenandoah pioneer cabin and get a glimpse of settlers' lifeways? And get there using a steep trail created and tramped well before Shenandoah was a national park? If you find the above appealing, here's something to sweeten the pot: Corbin Cabin is available for overnight rental by the public! Even if you don't spend the night, this is still a worthy destination. Not only is the cabin interesting, but the surrounding upper Hughes River is a naturally alluring locale. The brevity of the hike—1.4 miles each way—makes up for the thousand-foot elevation change. If you take your time going up or down, almost anyone can make it.

Best Time

This is a fine year-round destination. No matter what season, visiting the historic Corbin Cabin will give you insight into pre-park pioneer life. Even if the Hughes River is excessively high in spring, you can still see the cabin without having to make the crossing.

Finding the Trail

The Corbin Cabin Cutoff Trail is on the east side of Skyline Drive at milepost 37.9. The parking area has seven spaces and is on the west side of the road. The trailhead is on a hilly curve and is easily missed.

Trail Description

Leave the east side of Skyline Drive on the Corbin Cabin Cutoff Trail. ▶1 This path was not created

TRAIL USE
Dayhiking

LENGTH
2.8 miles, 2½–3½ hours

CUMULATIVE ELEVATION +/-
-1,020'/+1,020'

DIFFICULTY
– 1 2 **3** 4 5 +

TRAIL TYPE
Out & Back

START & FINISH
N38° 36.938'
W78° 21.052'

FEATURES
Ridgeline
Stream
Autumn Colors
Wildflowers
Historic Interest

FACILITIES
Rental cabin

Visit an intact authentic pioneer cabin.

▲ **Ridgeline**

🍁 **Autumn Colors**

🌸 **Wildflowers**

by park personnel but was simply beaten down by natives of these Potomac Highlands. The national park generally builds trails with a lesser gradient and takes into account several factors, such as minimizing erosion, stabilizing the trailbed, avoiding sensitive locations for flora and fauna, and routing toward scenic locales. Park personnel have since added waterbars, cleared trees, and strategically placed rocks to keep the trail from washing away.

Enter hardwoods of birch, striped maple, and oak. Grasses wave across the forest floor. Quickly join a rib ridge emanating from the crest of Shenandoah. Pines and mountain laurel increase in number on this xeric hilltop. Thorofare Mountain rises to your right, as does Stony Man Mountain.

The path steepens at 0.4 mile. It has to lose that elevation sooner or later. At 0.5 mile, the trail turns off the ridge and into a hollow. Reach the head of the hollow at 0.7 mile. ▶2 You are halfway. A trickling branch gurgles amid the rocks, falling to feed the Hughes River. Wildflowers grace the trailside in spring. Lots of rock piles scattered throughout the hollow are signs of cultivation, perhaps by George Corbin himself. Look also for rock walls and overgrown roads. At 1.2 miles, the trail comes alongside a conspicuous rock wall. Step over a little spring

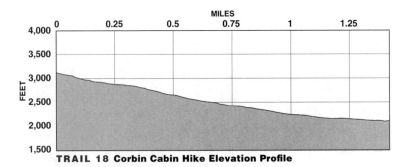

TRAIL 18 Corbin Cabin Hike Elevation Profile

branch. The woods are starting to flatten out some-what. Look right for a narrow path leading uphill to an old pioneer cemetery.

The Hughes River greets you with a watery song. Look to your right in a flat before the stream to see the remnants of a forgotten structure. Its floor and roof are still intact, but most of the walls have collapsed.

 Stream

Rock-hop the Hughes River. To your left, the Nicholson Hollow Trail has come up 4 miles from the community of Nethers. It leads right up to Skyline Drive. The Corbin Cabin stands in front of you, in a small clearing kept open to reduce the possibility of fire taking down the historic structure. ▶3 If it is unoccupied, the building will be closed tightly, but you still can take a seat on the porch to admire the view. The clearing opens to river, rock, and forest, all protected by national park status. Most pioneer cabins were dismantled, but luckily this one was spared for us to experience.

Historic Interest

When George Corbin built his two-story wood-and-chinking cabin on the banks of the upper Hughes River in 1910, deep in the Potomac Highlands of Virginia, he never imagined it would become a national park attraction on the National Register of Historic Places. Corbin lived in his cre-ation until 1938, when Shenandoah National Park bought him out and he moved outside the newly established boundaries. A legend persists that the cabin is haunted by George's wife Nee who died there during childbirth in the winter of 1924. If you are brave enough to stay, obtain more cabin rental information at **www.patc.net.**

🚶	**MILESTONES**	
▶1	0.0	Corbin Cabin parking area at milepost 37.9
▶2	0.7	Turn down the hollow toward Hughes River
▶3	1.4	Corbin Cabin

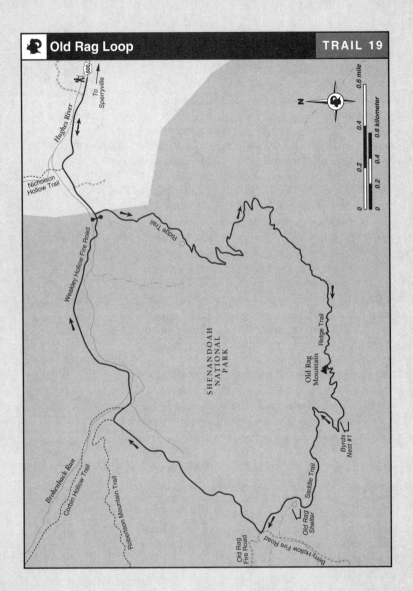

Old Rag Loop

TRAIL 19

To Sperryville

600

Hughes River

Nicholson Hollow Trail

Weakley Hollow Fire Road

Ridge Trail

SHENANDOAH NATIONAL PARK

Old Rag Mountain Ridge Trail

Byrds Nest #1

Brokenback Run

Corbin Hollow Trail

Robertson Mountain Trail

Saddle Trail

Old Rag Shelter

Old Rag Fire Road

Berry Hollow Fire Road

N

0.6 mile

0.6 kilometer

0.2   0.4

0   0.2   0.4

Old Rag Loop

Old Rag is Shenandoah National Park's addition to the great mountains of America. The granite-topped peak is the park's most recognizable and beloved—literally—summit. It is famed for its boulder scramble and the multiplicity of views from the rock protuberances adorning its flanks. And the Old Rag loop is a Shenandoah classic, a must-do feather in your hiking cap, but it is the most difficult hike in this entire guidebook. The rock scramble and the elevation gain have everything to do with this rating.

Despite the challenges, this hike is popular to the extreme. If there is any way, save your trek for a weekday. But hiking it on a weekend is better than not hiking it at all. Strike up the north slope of the mountain, then emerge onto a massive granite slab with incredible panoramas. Enter a maze of boulders, with some bona fide rock scrambling to reach the summit. The views are among the best in the park. Leave the rugged mountaintop, and reenter the lowlands along the pretty valley of Brokenback Run on a foot-relieving gravel fire road.

Best Time

This very busy hike is best done on clear, dry weekdays, not only to minimize crowding and maximize views, but also for safe hiking. The loop requires a challenging rock scramble that could become hazardous in wet or icy conditions. Also, be apprised pets are not allowed on half the hike, so please leave your dog at home on this trek.

TRAIL USE
Dayhiking,
Pets Prohibited

LENGTH
9.1 miles, 6–8 hours

**CUMULATIVE
ELEVATION +/-**
+2,425'/-2,425'

DIFFICULTY
– 1 2 3 4 **5** +

TRAIL TYPE
Loop

START & FINISH
N38° 34.297'
W78° 17.346'

FEATURES
Ridgeline
Stream
Summit
Autumn Colors
Wildflowers
Geologic Interest
Great Views

FACILITIES
Restrooms at trailhead

Finding the Trail

From the intersection of US 211 and US 522 in Sperryville, take US 522 south for 0.8 mile to VA 231. Turn right on VA 231 and follow it 8 miles to VA 601, Peola Mills Road. Turn right on VA 601, and follow it 0.3 mile, cross the Hughes River, then veer right, staying with VA 601. Stay with the blacktop as it becomes Nethers Road and leads up the Hughes River Valley to the lower Old Rag parking lot at 3.3 miles. Park here.

Alternate directions: From the intersection of US 29 Business and VA 231 in Madison, take VA 231 north for 12.4 miles to VA 602, Nethers Road. Follow VA 602, and stay with Nethers Road for a total of 3.4 miles from VA 231 to reach the lower parking lot.

Trail Description

The hike starts with a road walk. Leave the lower parking area ▶1 and walk up the pavement of quiet VA 600, passing the Nicholson Hollow Trail at 0.5 mile. Make the upper parking area at 0.8 mile. ▶2 Head left on the Ridge Trail, officially entering the national park. The climb innocently starts beneath cove hardwoods on a wide, uniform slope. Trailside

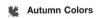 **Autumn Colors**

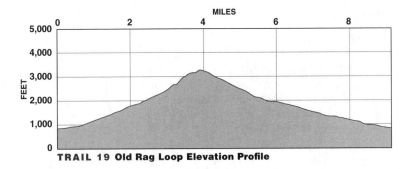

TRAIL 19 Old Rag Loop Elevation Profile

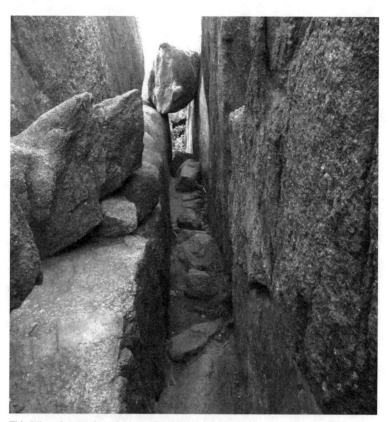

This hike *takes you through some tight squeezes.*

boulders give a hint of things to come. The path switchbacks a couple of times, then ascends along a small, boulder-strewn hollow. Sharply turn away from the hollow at 1.8 miles, rising through chestnut oaks, sassafras, and gum. More switchbacks diminish the slope's steepness. Pass a tiny rill at 2.5 miles. Still more switchbacks twist ahead. The trail levels off at 2.8 miles. Weary hikers rest at this point. The Ridge Trail turns sharply right, climbing more. Ascend onto a granite slab. Your initial panoramas open. ▶3

▲ **Ridgeline**

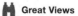 **Great Views**

Geologic Interest

The next mile is incredible, and incredibly challenging. Follow the blue blazes over, under, and around boulders, crevices, and outcrops. It takes both hands and feet across bare steep rock to achieve the peak. Intermittent wooded stretches break up the climb. It's challenging and exciting— you will use all fours. At times, the scramble seems like a grand, granite maze. Be careful and keep following the blue blazes painted on rock. Take your time to visit outlying granite openings to absorb views of the nearby summit you are scaling, the surrounding mountains, and the lowlands beyond.

Level off at 3.6 miles, on the rocky shoulder of Old Rag. More stone stands between you and the summit, which you reach at 3.9 miles. ▶4 A few rocks to your right create the high point at 3,268 feet. Wind-sculpted vegetation clings to life among the cracks and crevices. Certain areas are cordoned off to protect this vegetation. Find your favorite overlook and take a well-deserved break.

Summit

Great Views

Start down the Saddle Trail, which veers away from the peak through heavily canopied woodland. Make your way off the west slope of Old Rag, passing outcrops with views directly to Robertson Mountain. Reach stone Byrds Nest Shelter #1, located in a saddle, at 4.4 miles. ▶5 It is for day-use only, but would be convenient in a storm.

Continue switchbacking down in sharply sloped woods. Come to wooden Old Rag Shelter at 5.4 miles. ▶6 It is day-use only too. A short path leads to a reliable spring. Leave the shelter on a wide fire road. The easy hiking is a relief and contrasts completely with your ascent. Drift into a trail junction and gap filled with tall pines and hardwoods at 5.8 miles. ▶7 Turn right here, and head down the Weakley Hollow Fire Road.

After a sharp right on the fire road, you pass the Robertson Mountain Trail at 6.9 miles. Brokenback Run noisily cuts through the valley you have entered. Just past this intersection the Corbin Hollow Trail heads left. Keep straight, spanning Brokenback Run on a metal bridge at 7.1 miles. ►8 As you walk the road, look for the large, 18- to 24-inch leaves of the umbrella magnolia tree. The unmistakable leaves are pointed at both ends. This tree prefers low-elevation streamside environments. Look also for some huge rock piles from pioneer days.

Cross Brokenback Run again on three footbridges at 8.2 miles. Span a side stream on yet another footbridge, then complete the loop at the upper parking lot at 8.3 miles. ►9 From here, backtrack to the lower lot, completing the hike at 9.1 miles. ►10

 Stream

 Wildflowers

		MILESTONES
►1	0.0	Old Rag lower parking lot
►2	0.8	Reach upper parking lot for Old Rag, and turn left on Ridge Trail
►3	2.9	First vistas and rock scramble
►4	3.9	Old Rag summit and join Saddle Trail
►5	4.4	Byrds Nest Shelter #1
►6	5.4	Old Rag Shelter
►7	5.8	Right on Weakley Hollow Fire Road
►8	7.1	Cross Brokenback Run on a metal bridge
►9	8.3	Old Rag upper parking lot
►10	9.1	Old Rag lower parking lot

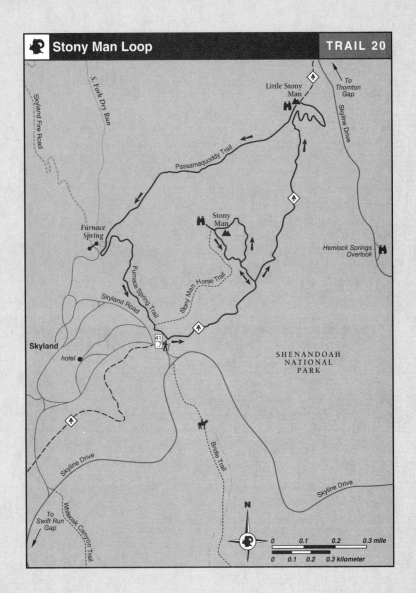

Stony Man Loop **TRAIL 20**

Little Stony
Man

S. Fork Dry Run

Skyland Fire Road

To
Thornton
Gap

Skyline Drive

Passamaquoddy Trail

Furnace
Spring

Stony
Man

Hemlock Springs
Overlook

Furnace Spring Trail

Skyland Road

Stony Man Horse Trail

Skyland

41
.7

hotel

SHENANDOAH
NATIONAL
PARK

Skyline Drive

Bridle Trail

Skyline Drive

To
Swift Run
Gap

Whiteoak Canyon Trail

N

0   0.1   0.2   0.3 mile

0   0.1   0.2   0.3 kilometer

Stony Man Loop

This hike traverses some of the highest terrain in the park. First you cruise a high-country nature trail and make a side loop to the summit of Stony Man Mountain, where cliffs rise 3,000 feet above the Shenandoah Valley and present superlative panoramas. You then take the Little Stony Man Trail to the peak of Little Stony Man, where more overlooks await. Your return trip is along the Passamaquoddy Trail, with still more views. Hike along the North Slope of Stony Man Mountain to reach Furnace Spring, which once was used in a copper mining operation. Climb through mixed evergreens and hardwoods back to the trailhead, completing this highlight-laden loop.

Best Time

This high-country hike will be cool even in summer. Yet you can best enjoy the views whenever the skies are clear, primarily spring and fall. Be apprised that the loop is busy on fair weather summer weekends.

Finding the Trail

This hike starts near the *north* entrance to Skyland Resort off Skyline Drive. At the turn you will see a sign indicating that this is the highest point on Skyline Drive. This turn is at milepost 41.7. Immediately after turning toward the Skyland Resort, turn right into the parking area for the Stony Man Nature Trail.

TRAIL USE
Dayhiking,
Pets Prohibited

LENGTH
3.4 miles, 2–3 hours

CUMULATIVE ELEVATION +/-
+800'/-800'

DIFFICULTY
– 1 2 **3** 4 5 +

TRAIL TYPE
Loop

START & FINISH
N38° 35.581'
W78° 22.548'

FEATURES
Ridgeline
Summit
Autumn Colors
Geologic Interest
Great Views
Historic Interest

FACILITIES
Nearby Skyland Resort

Trail Description

The beginning can be a little confusing. ▶1 Here a sign indicates the path as the Stony Man Nature Trail; however, this is also the Appalachian Trail (AT). They run in conjunction here. You can purchase an interpretive booklet at the trailhead to enhance your nature trail experience. Walk a pleasant pea-gravel path amid fern gardens overlain by hardwoods. Preserved hemlocks add a touch of evergreen to the woods. Later you will also see a few spruce trees.

At 0.4 mile, come to an intersection. ▶2 This is the highest point on the AT in Shenandoah National Park—3,837 feet. But you are fixing to get even higher. Turn left, still ascending to make the subloop to the summit of Stony Man, staying with the nature trail. Split right ahead, following the sequence of the interpretive posts. Note the squat, wind-sculpted haw trees as you climb.

At 0.7 mile, reach a four-way trail intersection. Turn right toward the summit of Stony Man. Incredible panoramas open ahead. ▶3 To your left, you can see the Skyland Resort. Ahead lay Shenandoah Valley and the town of Luray, Massanutten Mountain running parallel to the Blue Ridge, and beyond that North Mountain forming the Virginia-West Virginia state line. To your

🍁 Autumn Colors

▲ Ridgeline

🧍 Summit

🔭 Great Views

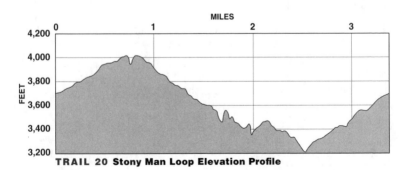

TRAIL 20 Stony Man Loop Elevation Profile

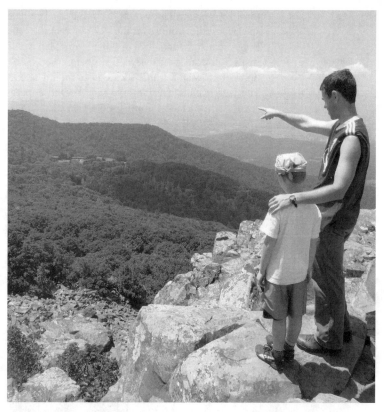

A father points out *Skyland and surrounding mountains in the distance from the crags of Stony Man.*

right, northerly, look below at the upthrust cliffs of Little Stony Man and at Skyline Drive and the park's north district. The name Stony Man derives from this peak—the park's second highest point—looking like the face of a bearded man. The Stony Man's face can be clearly seen from the north on milepost 38.9 of Skyline Drive at Stony Man Mountain Overlook.

Return to the Appalachian Trail, then resume a northbound direction. The trail drops steadily through northern hardwoods, including cool climate specialist yellow birch, on the east slope of the Blue Ridge. Reach the tan cliffs of Little Stony Man at 1.7 miles. ▶4 More grand views open before you. Look up to Stony Man for little stick figures milling about. The jagged cliffs have an especially rugged appearance as they emerge from the surrounding forest. The squared-off fields of Shenandoah Valley below contrast with the craggy mountains to your right.

Return to woods beyond the cliff, switchbacking downhill to make another trail junction at 1.9 miles. ▶5 Leave the white-blazed AT, and turn left on the Passamaquoddy Trail, blazed in blue. Soon pass beneath the cliffs of Little Stony Man on a path constructed with considerable effort from native stones. Open onto a lower outcrop that avails yet another overlook from which the west side of the Blue Ridge and Lake Arrowhead opens below. The rising slope of Stony Man Mountain is especially impressive. Begin meandering the northwest side of the peak on a steep slope, yet the well-constructed trail makes hiking a breeze. Walk beneath cliffs. Come to a rock overhang and dripping spring at 2.4 miles. At 2.5 miles, reach your low point of 3,200 feet, then begin a gentle uptick. Fire cherry trees are rising where hemlocks once stood. Pass beneath a transmission line at 2.8 miles.

Reach Furnace Spring at 2.9 miles. ▶6 You can hear the water flowing behind a locked door. The old copper mine was in this vicinity and used the spring, but the shaft has since been filled in and no trail leads to it. Come to an intersection with Skyland Fire Road and the Furnace Spring Trail. Make a hard left here, joining the yellow-blazed Furnace Spring Trail, passing directly above Furnace Spring on a double-track. The path then narrows and reenters deep woods. Snake your way uphill in rocky forest. The trailbed is fainter here. Look for yellow blazes on the trailside trees amid

Summit

Great Views

Wildflowers

Geologic Interest

Historic Interest

more preserved hemlocks. Meet the Stony Man Horse Trail, and turn left, tracing it a short distance to reach the Stony Man Nature Trail parking area and the hike's conclusion. ▶7

🚶 MILESTONES

▶1	0.0	Stony Man Nature Trail parking area at milepost 41.7
▶2	0.4	Left toward Stony Man Summit
▶3	0.8	Stony Man Summit
▶4	1.7	Little Stony Man Summit
▶5	1.9	Passamaquoddy Trail
▶6	2.9	Left on Furnace Spring Trail
▶7	3.4	Stony Man Nature Trail parking area at milepost 41.7

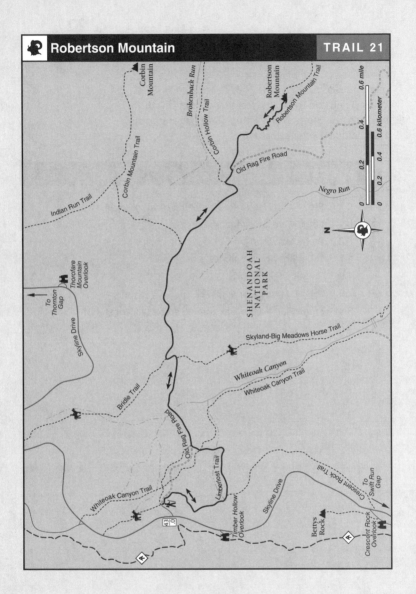

Robertson Mountain

Robertson Mountain is one of the park's better, but least visited, scenic summits. Reaching the rocky summit is neither difficult nor time-consuming, but most people pass it by to climb nearby Old Rag, one of the park's busiest destinations. But first you get to explore a highland cove and wetland on the all-access Limberlost Trail. You then join Old Rag Fire Road, where the walking is easy. A more traditional single-track foot trail takes you the last mile to the outcrops of Robertson Mountain. There, various rocky points avail sweeping views in three directions. The crowds thin out when you leave the Limberlost Trail, which offers an excellent short nature walk of 1.3 miles for anybody, even wheelchair-bound park enthusiasts.

Best Time

The trek to the outcrops on Robertson Mountain can be enjoyed most when the skies are clear.

Finding the Trail

The Limberlost Trail parking area is at milepost 43 on Skyline Drive. The signed parking area is just a short distance down a road on the east side of Skyline Drive. It is 12.5 miles south of the Thornton Gap Entrance Station on Skyline Drive.

Trail Description

To begin, take the gravelly Limberlost Trail right from the parking area, ▶1 and enter a former

TRAIL USE
Dayhiking
LENGTH
6.8 miles, 3½–5 hours
CUMULATIVE ELEVATION +/-
-1,080'/+1,080'
DIFFICULTY
– 1 2 3 **4 5** +
TRAIL TYPE
Out & Back
START & FINISH
N38° 34.805'
W78° 22.879'

FEATURES
Stream
Ridgeline
Summit
Autumn Colors
Great Views

FACILITIES
None

hemlock forest that Skyland Resort founder George Freeman Pollock helped protect nearly a century ago. *Be apprised that the Limberlost Trail is closed to pets.* Unfortunately the hemlock woolly adelgid did in most of the hemlocks, though a few are preserved. White oaks, yellow birch, mountain laurel, and even some apple trees round out the forest mosaic. Ferns carpet moister areas in the cool perched valley standing higher than 3,200 feet. The pea-gravel track gently meanders through this upper drainage of Whiteoak Run. Contemplation benches have been placed astride the path.

At 0.4 mile, traverse a boardwalk spanning an upland marsh. ▶2 Just ahead, the Crescent Rock Trail leaves right. Stay straight with the Limberlost Trail, passing through a former hemlock grove now being supplanted by bushy pin cherry trees. These transitional cherries will shade climax species, such as yellow birch, red spruce, and maybe hemlock when the forest reaches its full glory again, long after our lifetimes. At 0.8 mile, bridge a tributary of Whiteoak Run. At 0.9 mile, reach a four-way junction. ▶3 Here, the Whiteoak Canyon Trail leaves right for the cavalcade of cataracts that characterizes its lower reaches.

Stay straight with the Limberlost Trail, shortly meeting Old Rag Fire Road. Turn right onto the

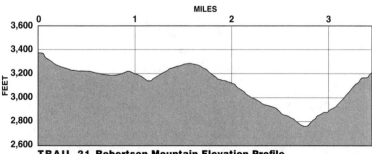

TRAIL 21 Robertson Mountain Elevation Profile

yellow-blazed fire road where a sign reads, "Horse Path, Skyland, Big Meadows." ▶4 The wide gravel track drops easterly, bridging Whiteoak Run at 1.1 miles. Stay left at a road split just ahead—this is where the horse concessionaire at Skyland turns around. The fire road climbs away from the stream to reach a trail junction at 1.4 miles. Stay left on Old Rag Fire Road. Just ahead, when a horse trail leads left, stay right. At 1.6 miles, you pass an old ranger station turned maintenance building on your right. ▶5

> ▶ **Stream**

> ▲ **Ridgeline**

Begin a protracted downgrade. Watch for size-able oak trees scattered amid the woods. The trail turns sharply to the left and approaches the Corbin Mountain Trail at 2.2 miles. ▶6 Keep descending gently on Old Rag Fire Road past more big trees.

Pass Corbin Hollow Trail at 2.7 miles. ▶7 Begin looking for the blue-blazed Robertson Mountain Trail ahead, where you turn left at 2.8 miles. ▶8 Your descent is over. The serpentine footpath, contrasting with the gentle nature trail and the wide fire road, enters a laurel thicket and then turns back right. Look for the huge oak tree at the turn. You curve around the green giant. It would take three hikers with arms outstretched to encircle it.

The real climbing doesn't start for another quarter mile, where the path switchbacks among rocks and trees, crowded by mountain laurel. It is hard to figure out which way the trail is going—except up. At 3.3 miles, the trail passes the summit on your right. Look on your right for a blue-blazed spur trail to the peak. The balance of the Robertson Mountain Trail leads straight. Take the spur past a grassy flat, ideal for picnicking, then continue on to the highest of several outcrops on Robertson Mountain. ▶9

> ▟ **Summit**

The depths of Whiteoak Canyon fall below. Look for the cleared overlooks along Skyline Drive and the Blue Ridge. The hump of Hawksbill Mountain looms tall to the southwest. Views to the north are

Great Views

a little harder to find, but scout around. Old Rag is to the east. Interestingly, Robertson Mountain, at 3,296 feet, is five feet higher than Old Rag. Take your time to take it all in; scout for more outcrops. It's great being on top of this mountain. On your return trip, near the trailhead, you can backtrack on the Limberlost Trail or take Old Rag Fire Road directly to the parking area.

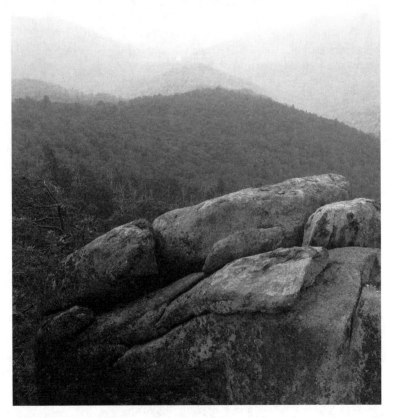

One of the many outcrops *that provide views of Robertson Mountain*

MILESTONES

▶1	0.0	Limberlost Trail parking area
▶2	0.4	Crescent Rock Trail leaves right
▶3	0.9	Bisect Whiteoak Canyon Trail
▶4	1.0	Right on Old Rag Fire Road
▶5	1.6	Pass old ranger station on right
▶6	2.2	Corbin Mountain Trail leaves left
▶7	2.7	Corbin Hollow Trail leaves left
▶8	2.8	Left on Robertson Mountain Trail
▶9	3.4	Robertson Mountain summit

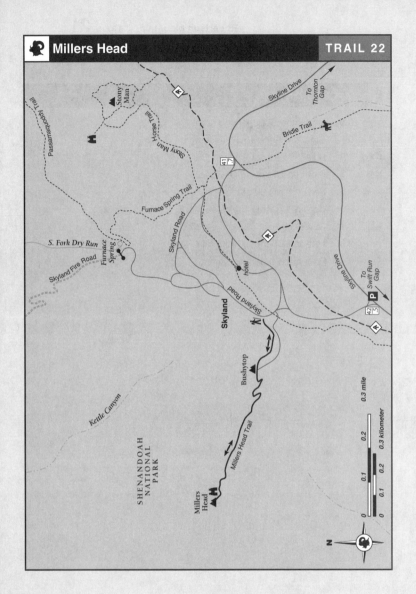

Stony Man

Passamaquoddy Trail

Stony Man Horse Trail

Skyline Drive

To Thornton Gap

Bridle Trail

41
7

R

Furnace Spring Trail

R

S. Fork Dry Run

Skyland Road

Skyland Fire Road

Furnace Spring

hotel

Skyline Drive

To Swift Run Gap

P

22
15

R

Skyland

Skyland Road

Bushytop

Kettle Canyon

Millers Head Trail

SHENANDOAH
NATIONAL
PARK

Millers
Head

0   0.1   0.2   0.3 mile

0   0.1   0.2   0.3 kilometer

N

Millers Head

This walk stretches west on a narrow ridge from the crest of greater Stony Man Mountain, the natural centerpiece where George Freeman Pollock owned 5,300 acres and developed his Skyland Resort, begun in 1890. Today's lodge guests often use the Millers Head Trail for short nature walks and sunset treks, to view the onset of night as the sun descends over the Allegheny Mountains to the west. Start high, adjacent to lodge facilities, and surmount a wooded knob to enjoy the view from Bushy Head. From there, you wind westerly, passing a wonderful view from an unnamed outcrop. At the trail's end, a stone platform allows widespread westerly panoramas from the bottom of Shenandoah Valley to West Virginia and points between.

The immediate history of the area not only encompasses Skyland Resort, but also the establishment of park facilities. The very first Civilian Conservation Corps (CCC) work camp in a national park was situated at Skyland. Freeman had pledged his land to the park, and thus it was chosen to develop national park facilities. At this point, in 1933, only the corridor of Skyline Drive had been authorized by the U.S. Congress, so park work at that point was limited to a strip adjacent to Skyline Drive. Later, when Shenandoah National Park was established in 1935, CCC camps and their projects spread throughout the park.

George Freeman Pollock was a notorious promoter of his Skyland Resort and worked for the establishment of Shenandoah National Park with equal zeal. His father came upon the Stony Man property as part of a mining claim that extracted

TRAIL USE
Dayhiking,
Child-Friendly

LENGTH
1.4 miles, 1–2 hours

CUMULATIVE
ELEVATION +/-
-290'/-290'

DIFFICULTY
− 1 **2** 3 4 5 +

TRAIL TYPE
Out & Back

START & FINISH
N38° 35.464'
W78° 23.026'

FEATURES
Ridgeline
Autumn Colors
Great Views

FACILITIES
Nearby Skyland Resort

copper from the mountain. Young George saw not a mine but a place to escape the heat of the Virginia summer, a place to relax in a beautiful natural setting. He sold cabin lots and later built dining and recreation halls on the property. Twelve of the original pre-park Skyland buildings remain. It is easy to visualize visitors from a century back, walking to the view at Millers Head.

Best Time

This hike is best when the skies are their most clear—spring, fall, and on dry winter days.

Finding the Trail

There is no parking at the Millers Head Trail beginning. You must park at the upper Whiteoak Canyon Trailhead, at Skyline Drive milepost 42.5, near the southern entrance to Skyland Resort complex, which adds 0.4 mile each way for whoever parks the car.

However, you can drop off part of your crew at the Millers Head Trailhead near the park amphitheater at Skyland. To reach it turn into the southern Skyland entrance at milepost 42.5, passing horse stable parking and continuing straight. At 0.3 mile veer left on the road toward the amphitheater. The

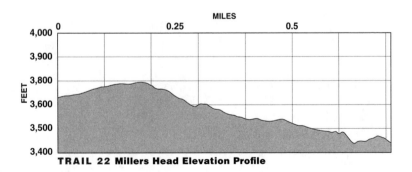

TRAIL 22 Millers Head Elevation Profile

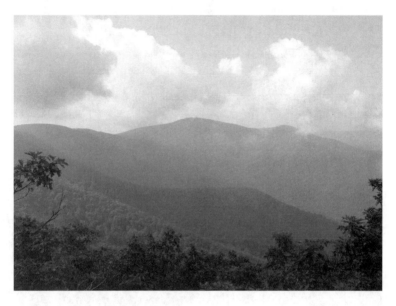

Looking south *to Hawksbill from Millers Head Trail*

left turn has a "No Outlet" sign. Walk just past the amphitheater, and you will see the Millers Head Trailhead in a small grassy area on the left, across the road from the Franklin building of greater Skyland Resort.

Trail Description

Join the hiking trail in a locust grove mixed with apple trees on the edge of a meadow. ▶1 Note the windswept branches of the trees on this highland locale. The dirt and rock path wanders uphill into a forest mosaic of preserved hemlocks, oaks, and maples, even some yellow birch. At 0.1 mile an old road leaves left, and you keep climbing to reach a communication building at 0.2 mile. ▶2 It is all downhill from here. Begin your downgrade to shortly meet a concrete signpost. Here, a short spur

 Autumn Colors

How the CCC Transformed Shenandoah

The Great Depression hit the United States in 1929, following a devastating stock market crash. At the time, no one knew how long the economic hard times would go on. In 1933, with the country still in the throes of economic malaise, President Franklin Delano Roosevelt initiated a government work program, the Civilian Conservation Corps, commonly known as the CCC. Through the program, men were hired on various projects throughout the United States, including transforming Shenandoah into the park we see today.

To qualify for the CCC, recruits had to be between the ages of 17 and 25, be out of school, and be unemployed. Eligible enrollees were often shipped far from homes to prevent desertion. They earned $30 per month for their efforts, of which $25 went back home. They built hiking trails, scenic roads, cabins, dams, and fish hatcheries; improved wildlife habitat; planted trees; and more at more than 800 parks in the United States.

The CCC was organized into camps, generally of 100 to 300 men, using a military structure with an emphasis on discipline. Each camp had its specialists, from cooks to officers. Camp life was routine. The men generally rose around 6 a.m., ate a filling breakfast, and then worked until 4:30 in the afternoon, with a lunch break in the middle. Whether the CCC helped or hurt the nation's economy remains under debate. The CCC program continued until 1942, when potential enrollees instead entered the military to fight World War II. Most of the CCC boys have passed away, but their legacy lives on here at Shenandoah.

Great Views

goes right to an outcrop and view known as Bushy Head. It presents westerly warm-up views of Kettle Canyon and the Shenandoah Valley. None other than George Freeman Pollock's ashes were scattered to the winds from this point, back in 1951. Thank ol' George for his work in making this national park a reality.

Continue descending on a rock track winding down the ridge via switchbacks. Lichen-covered boulders and hardwoods flank the path. Dip to a gap at 0.4 mile. The trees become more stunted as you extend farther out on this peninsula. At 0.5 mile, a short trail leads left to an outcrop and a vista to the south. ▶3 The view stretches across Timber Hollow. The highest point you can see is the highest point in Shenandoah National Park—Hawksbill.

Descend to cut through another gap in the ridge. The trail curves around the north side of the ridge amid ferns aplenty; the crest is bouldery to the extreme. Return to the ridgecrest, and walk a bit more to emerge onto the stone platform of Millers Head. ▶4 To the left you can see Skyline Drive and Hawksbill. The town of Luray stands in the foreground backed by Massanutten Mountain. To the right is more of Stony Man Mountain, if the view has been recently cleared. A still listener will hear sounds of civilization drifting up from the valley more than 2,500 feet below.

▲ **Ridgeline**

🔭 **Great Views**

🔭 **Great Views**

🚶	**MILESTONES**		
▶1	0.0	Millers Head Trail near Skyland Amphitheater
▶2	0.2	Bushy Head
▶3	0.5	View of Hawksbill to left of trail
▶4	0.7	Millers Head Overlook

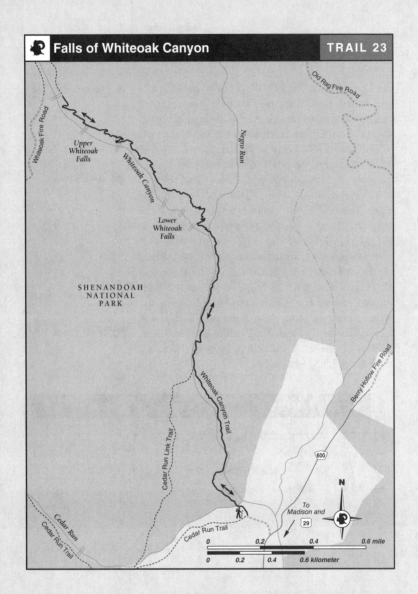

Falls of Whiteoak Canyon — **TRAIL 23**

Old Rag Fire Road

Whiteoak Fire Road

Upper Whiteoak Falls

Whiteoak Canyon

Negro Run

Lower Whiteoak Falls

SHENANDOAH NATIONAL PARK

Cedar Run Link Trail

Whiteoak Canyon Trail

Berry Hollow Fire Road

600

N

To Madison and 29

Cedar Run

Cedar Run Trail

Cedar Run Trail

| 0 | 0.2 | 0.4 | 0.6 mile |

| 0 | 0.2 | 0.4 | 0.6 kilometer |

Falls of Whiteoak Canyon

It's hard to keep track of all the falls at Whiteoak Canyon. There are six sequentially numbered falls. The count starts from the Blue Ridge and ends at the base of the canyon. To confuse matters further, this hike starts at the bottom of Whiteoak Run and heads upstream. Whether or not you correctly identify and number the falls, take this classic Shenandoah hike, for there are not only falls but also canyon views and everywhere-you-look beauty. However, beware the warm weather weekend crowds. I highly recommend heading in a different direction during these times.

Best Time

Since this hike has no fords, you can hike it in winter and spring without worry. That's when the falls are their boldest. In spring, wildflowers are their showiest. By all means avoid this crowded hike on summer and fall weekends with nice weather.

Finding the Trail

From the town of Madison, on US 29 north of Charlottesville and south of Culpepper, drive north on VA 231 for 5 miles to VA 670. Turn left on VA 670, and follow it for 5 miles to VA 643. Turn right on VA 643, and follow it for less than a mile to VA 600. Turn left on VA 600, and follow it for 3.7 miles to Berry Hollow. The trailhead is in the back of the far parking area, which is on your right.

TRAIL USE
Dayhiking

LENGTH
5.2 miles, 3½–4½ hours

CUMULATIVE ELEVATION +/-
+1,400'/-1,400'

DIFFICULTY
– 1 2 3 **4** 5 +

TRAIL TYPE
Out & Back

START & FINISH
N38° 32.370'
W78° 20.962'

FEATURES
Stream
Waterfalls
Wildflowers
Geologic Interest
Great Views
Steep

FACILITIES
None

Trail Description

Leave the rear of the parking area in Whiteoak Canyon, ►1 and travel a trail easement through private property, reaching Cedar Run. At this point, the streambed is often dry, even though Cedar Run may be flowing upstream. Span Cedar Run on a metal bridge. Beech, sycamore, black birch, and magnolia shade the track. Ferns reflect the moist nature of a valley that is wide at this point and hasn't yet narrowed into a canyon.

Waterfall lovers: Don't miss this hike.

 Stream

When you reach the Cedar Run Trail junction at mile 0.2, ►2 veer right, staying on the Whiteoak Canyon Trail. The Cedar Run Trail leads left for its own series of falls on an ultra-rocky path. Bridge Whiteoak Run, a rocky river if there ever was one. The sandy trail gently ascends along the right bank of the creek. Sycamores overhang the stream. The rock walls and piles are evidence that this area was once cultivated.

Come directly alongside the stream and reach the junction with the Cedar Run Link Trail at 0.8 mile. ►3 Backcountry camping is prohibited beyond this point. Beyond here, the terrain is steep and rocky and not suitable for pitching a tent. Stay on the east bank of Whiteoak Run, entering a rock garden. The canyon closes. The

 Wildflowers

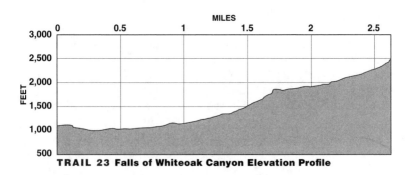

TRAIL 23 Falls of Whiteoak Canyon Elevation Profile

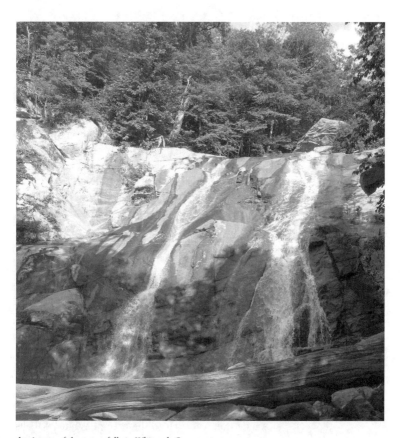

Just one *of the many falls in Whiteoak Canyon*

stream begins gathering in deep pools. The path becomes correspondingly rockier and steeper. Rock-hop Negro Run, which has a falls of its own, on your right. Just beyond this crossing, close in on Lower Whiteoak Falls (number six) at 1.4 miles. ►4 A short trail leads left to the precipitous two-tier, 60-foot falls, which spills over an open rock face. The uppermost falls, where this hike ends, is the canyon's tallest at 86 feet. The ones in between—that are hard to count because their tops

Waterfall

and bottoms are indiscernible—purportedly range between 45 and 65 feet each.

The main trail switchbacks, meandering far away from the stream. The area can be confusing because erosive user-created trails continue straight up the canyon. Follow the switchbacks on the proper trail. Climb sharply along the base of a bluff in pines, well above the stream, sometimes traversing open rock. In places, steps have been chiseled into this bare stone. At 1.7 miles, come to a cedar tree that guards a rock slab overlook into the canyon. Catch glimpses of the crashing falls below and the lands beyond the canyon. Continue switchbacking up the canyon and below other cliffs. The stream and path come together again by 1.9 miles. This is where the numbered falls get confusing. Just enjoy the cataracts and leave the counting to others.

Begin a pattern of coming to a falls and then switchbacking away and uphill to the base of another falls. Huge walls rise beyond the stream. Pass an overhanging boulder on your right at 2.3 miles. Keep climbing through a wonderment of rock and water, where pools and cascades beckon you off the trail and to Whiteoak Run.

As you continue uphill, a melding of stone and concrete makes the pathway more hiker-friendly. A side trail leads left to the base of Whiteoak Falls (number one) at 2.4 miles. ▶5 The main trail switchbacks to the right and passes a concrete trail marker indicating the halfway point of the Whiteoak Canyon Trail, with an attendant warning for hikers that a shuttle is unavailable at the bottom of the canyon. Apparently, hikers have walked the Whiteoak Canyon Trail from Skyline Drive and decided they couldn't walk back up. Come to a rock observation point for Whiteoak Canyon Falls (number one) at 2.6 miles. ▶6 You are on a large slab well above the second highest falls in the park at 86 feet. It slides over bare rock in multiple stages bordered by

Steep

Great Views

Waterfall

Waterfall

hardwoods. Rest and enjoy these falls and the good view into the canyon below. On your return trip try to count the falls. After all, Whiteoak Run has more falls per mile than any other stream in the park.

		MILESTONES
▶1	0.0	Whiteoak Canyon Trailhead
▶2	0.2	Cedar Run Trail leaves left
▶3	0.8	Cedar Run Link Trail leaves left
▶4	1.4	Lower Whiteoak Canyon Falls (number six)
▶5	2.4	Side trail to base of uppermost Whiteoak Canyon Falls (number one)
▶6	2.6	Whiteoak Canyon Falls (number one) observation point

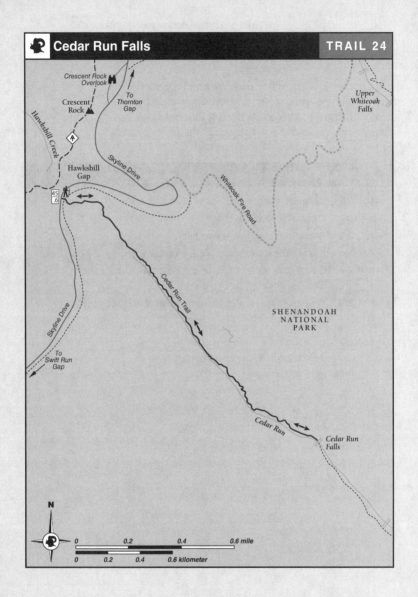

Crescent Rock
Overlook

To
Thornton
Gap

Crescent
Rock

Upper
Whiteoak
Falls

Hawksbill Creek

Skyline Drive

Hawksbill
Gap

45
6

Whiteoak Fire Road

Cedar Run Trail

SHENANDOAH
NATIONAL
PARK

Skyline Drive

To
Swift Run
Gap

Cedar Run

Cedar Run
Falls

N

0   0.2   0.4   0.6 mile
0   0.2   0.4   0.6 kilometer

Cedar Run Falls

This hike leads you into rugged upper Cedar Run Canyon. The trail down to the falls is steep as it passes innumerable cascades spilling down the narrow boulder-laden gorge. This place is wild and deserving of national park protection. Your trip to the cascades will be slow because you need to watch your footing and stop often to admire the scenery.

Best Time

The falls are their boldest during winter and spring. Also, spring has flowers galore. More important, avoid this busy hike on nice weekends any time of year.

Finding the Trail

The Hawksbill Gap Trailhead is located at milepost 45.6 on Skyline Drive. The Cedar Run Trail starts behind the gravel parking area on the east side of Skyline Drive.

Trail Description

Leave the parking area and grassy Hawksbill Gap behind to enter tall hardwoods on the Cedar Run Trail. ▶1 Immediately come to a four-way trail junction. Keep forward, descending, still on the Cedar Run Trail. The Skyland-Big Meadows Horse Trail leaves left and right. Pass a rock outcrop often used as a relaxing locale for those returning up Cedar Run Canyon. The trail grade drops sharply in a thick forest alongside the upper reaches of Cedar Run. Step over rock and wood waterbars that cut down on trail

TRAIL USE
Dayhiking

LENGTH
3.4 miles, 3–4 hours

CUMULATIVE ELEVATION +/-
-1,475'/+1,475'

DIFFICULTY
– 1 2 3 **4** 5 +

TRAIL TYPE
Out & Back

START & FINISH
N38° 33.363'
W78° 23.197'

FEATURES
Stream
Autumn Colors
Wildflowers
Geologic Interest
Waterfalls
Steep

FACILITIES
None

 Steep

169

erosion. The white noise of cold mountain water serenades you all the way to the falls.

A northern hardwood forest of cherry, witch hazel, sugar maple, and large oaks rise from the stony woods. Despite elaborate trail work by the park service, the path remains very rocky. Take your time and carefully plant your feet—a rolled ankle is possible here. Sturdy boots and trekking poles will make the Cedar Run Trail more palatable. On the plus side: The plethora of boulders avails for ample resting spots on your return trip.

Cedar Run picks up steam on its drop, falling in multiple incarnations of moving water. A side branch crosses the trail, forming a cascade of its own. Soon, you walk alongside the fast-moving run. At 0.6 mile, step onto a wide rock, facing a cascade to your right. ▶2 Cedar Run descends 20 feet in a fan pattern and then crashes onto the rock on which you are standing.

Beyond this cascade the trail drops steeply alongside a stair-step cascade to your right and a rocky bluff to your left. At 0.9 mile, enjoy a brief interlude of level, relatively rock-free pathway. Then the trail resumes diving headlong into a cavalcade of stone and passes another slide cascade. At other times monstrous midstream boulders nearly obscure the water as it seeks gravity's level. At 1.1

Autumn Colors

Stream

Waterfall

Wildflowers

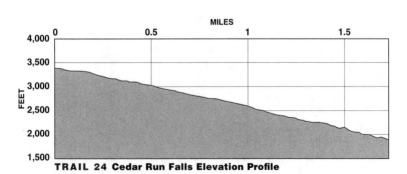

TRAIL 24 Cedar Run Falls Elevation Profile

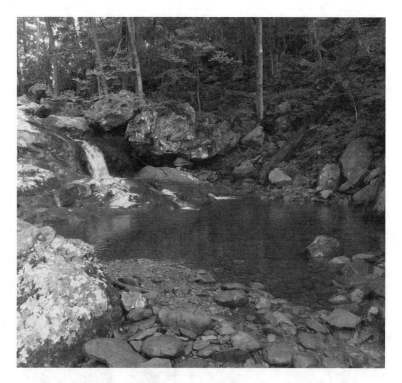

Rock and water *combine to create scenes like this one in Cedar Run Canyon.*

miles, away from the stream, rock ramparts rise from the trees, forming canyon walls that echo and redouble the sounds of moving water. ▶3

At 1.3 miles, on the far side of the trail, a tributary stream adds its flow in a slide cascade. A deep pool with brook trout forms on Cedar Run just below this tributary. The clash of water and rock remains relentless. At 1.4 miles, pass another cliff line. ▶4 At 1.5 miles, the trail comes to a big, alluring pool below a two-tier cascade. ▶5 You have reached the crossing of Cedar Run. This is usually a rock-hop; however, it can be a wet crossing at high water.

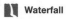 Waterfall

Discover a wild, rocky canyon deserving of park protection.

Waterfall

Geologic Interest

You are now on the right-hand bank heading downstream. Yet the trail goes uphill, passing a feeder stream trickling in from your right. The Cedar Run Trail then descends a set of stone steps to the base of Cedar Run Falls at 1.7 miles. ▶6 The water spills down a slick rock face and lands in a deep and clear plunge pool, then it drops again in a whitewater froth through a narrow slot canyon. Many large boulders make good relaxing and observation points at this mid-falls area. Half Mile Cliff rises on the far side of the falls.

You can go a bit farther downstream to enjoy the lower segment of Cedar Run Falls. It has a deep

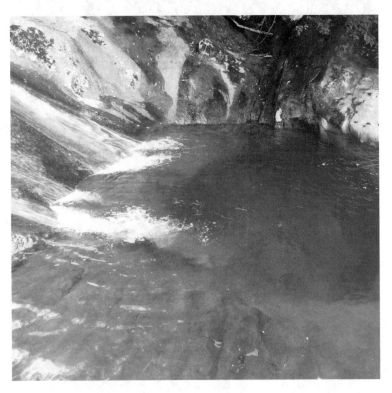

A clear pool *lies at the base of the falls on Cedar Run.*

plunge pool at the base of the slot canyon. You'll likely think of reasons to hang out down here since the hike back is ambitious (i.e., very steep). Pace yourself, and use those trailside boulders to catch some air.

🚶	**MILESTONES**	
▶1	0.0	Hawksbill Gap parking area at milepost 45.6
▶2	0.6	Wide cascade
▶3	1.1	Trailside cliff line
▶4	1.4	Trailside cliff line
▶5	1.5	Cross Cedar Run
▶6	1.7	Cedar Run Falls

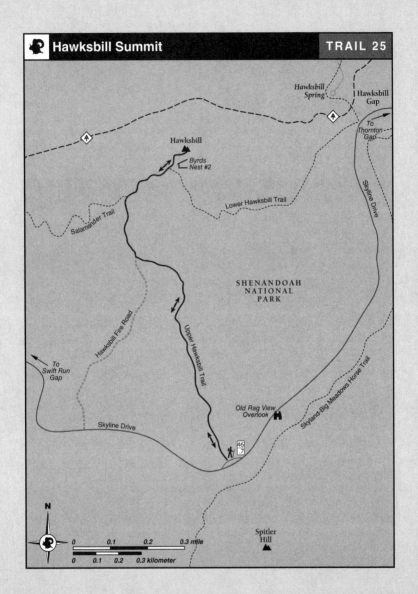

Hawksbill Spring

Hawksbill Gap

To Thornton Gap

Hawksbill

Byrds Nest #2

Lower Hawksbill Trail

Salamander Trail

Skyline Drive

SHENANDOAH NATIONAL PARK

Hawksbill Fire Road

Upper Hawksbill Trail

To Swift Run Gap

Old Rag View Overlook

Skyland-Big Meadows Horse Trail

46
.7

Skyline Drive

N

0   0.1   0.2   0.3 mile

0   0.1   0.2   0.3 kilometer

Spitler Hill

Hawksbill Summit

This is an easy, favorite hike that starts at a high elevation and gets to the top of things in Shenandoah. Along the way you enter a "sky island" of Canadian-type forest. Outcrops below the summit are just warm-ups for the nearly 360-degree view from the summit of Hawksbill.

Best Time

Whenever the skies are clear is a good time to make Hawksbill. Since it is the park's highest point, Hawksbill receives heavy visitation, especially during summer.

Finding the Trail

The Upper Hawksbill Trailhead is on the west side of Skyline Drive at milepost 46.7. From the Thornton Gap Entrance Station, take Skyline Drive south for 15.2 miles to reach the parking area, on your right.

Trail Description

You get a jump on bagging this peak by starting out at higher than 3,600 feet, leaving less than 500 feet of vertical gain to the nose of Hawksbill. Leave from the back of the Upper Hawksbill parking area on the wide and gravelly Upper Hawksbill Trail. ▶1 Upland hardwoods of oak, birch, and maples line the track. Look for a few preserved hemlocks in the forest. Note how their lowermost branches grow

TRAIL USE
Dayhiking

LENGTH
2.2 miles, 1½–2 hours

CUMULATIVE ELEVATION +/-
+415'/-415'

DIFFICULTY
− 1 **2** 3 4 5 +

TRAIL TYPE
Out & Back

START & FINISH
N38° 32.615'
W78° 23.591'

FEATURES
Summit
Autumn Colors
Great Views

FACILITIES
None

🍁 **Autumn Colors**

in a ring of uniform height. This is a result of deer browsing—they can reach only so far up the tree, leaving this halo of greenery. The trail makes a quick jump and continues at a moderate grade. The small logs or waterbars across the trailbed help prevent erosion during prolonged rains and thunderstorms that sometimes wrack the Blue Ridge.

At this elevation the growing season is short; the trees don't begin to foliate until later May. Late September finds leaves turning a kaleidoscope of colors as trees prepare for a cold season that's significantly longer than that in the adjoining valleys. At 0.4 mile, the trail levels off then actually descends to reach the Hawksbill Fire Road at 0.6 mile. ▶2

Turn right and head up the gullied fire road, a wider track than the one you've been traveling. Begin to look for Fraser fir and red spruce, two northern climate species that are rare in Shenandoah and the Old Dominion. The evergreens are components of the Canadian-type (or boreal) forest that covered much of Shenandoah thousands of years ago. As the climate warmed and the ancient glaciers receded, these trees clung to the highest peaks of the Appalachians, where it was still cool enough for them to survive, forming "sky islands" of these Canadian plant communities.

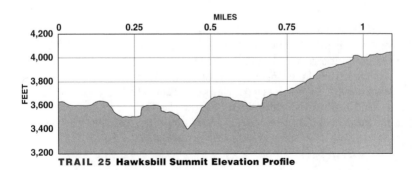

TRAIL 25 Hawksbill Summit Elevation Profile

At 0.9 mile, the Salamander Trail leaves left, and connects to the Appalachian Trail. ▶3 The main route to Hawksbill keeps straight and intersects the Lower Hawksbill Trail at 1.0 mile. ▶4 It leaves right for Hawksbill Gap. It seems that about everything in this vicinity is named Hawksbill.

Just ahead, come to a day-use shelter, Byrds Nest #2. It is a three-sided stone shelter, facing northwest. The refuge has a picnic table inside but the fireplace has been bricked shut. Camping is prohibited on the upper part of Hawksbill Mountain. The long, open rock promontory of the mountain— the hawk's bill—stretches in both directions from the shelter and offers a natural viewing deck.

 Summit

The main trail leaves right from the shelter. Ascend briefly and step up onto the Hawksbill (4,050 feet). ▶5 Though the exposed rocks provide good overlooks, the manmade observation platform, bordered by a decorative stone wall may help you orient yourself. Metal plates showing the cardinal points are laid into the rock walls of the platform. You are standing atop the highest point in Shenandoah National Park. And what views you'll find: Old Rag in the eastern distance, Stony Man to the north, Skyline Drive and Crescent Rock nearby, and Nakedtop, as well as towns and hollows in the Shenandoah Valley to the west. Take some time to walk along the rock rim, grabbing other views from other lookouts. It's a good feeling—being on top of the Blue Ridge.

 Great Views

🚶	MILESTONES	
▶1	0.0	Upper Hawksbill Trailhead at milepost 46.7
▶2	0.6	Right on Hawksbill Fire Road
▶3	0.9	Salamander Trail leaves left; stay right
▶4	1.0	Hawksbill Trail leaves right to Hawksbill Gap Trailhead
▶5	1.1	Hawksbill Summit at 4,050 feet

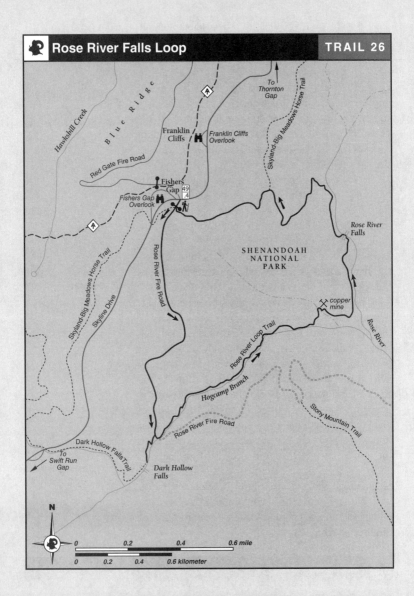

Rose River Falls Loop

This loop hike is long on beauty but sometimes short on solitude. Begin your trek on Rose River Fire Road, and gently descend to reach the lower Dark Hollow Falls Trail. Make the worthwhile 0.2-mile ascent to reach Dark Hollow Falls, while seeing other falls along this creek, Hogcamp Branch. Next, follow the Rose River Loop Trail downstream, passing numerous cascades along what is arguably the prettiest stream in the park. Bridge Hogcamp Branch, then pass the tailings of an old copper mine. Beyond here, the hike ascends the upper Rose River, passing Rose River Falls before returning to the trailhead.

Best Time

During spring the falls flow and the wildflowers grow. Summer and fall can be crowded. Hogcamp Branch, one stream along which you walk, can be a frozen delight in winter.

Finding the Trail

The Rose River Fire Road starts on the east side of Skyline Drive, just north of Fishers Gap Overlook at milepost 49.4. The parking is on the west side of the drive. The overlook is on a short, spur loop that leaves Skyline Drive. The Rose River Fire Road starts across Skyline Drive from the overlook's north end. From the Swift Run Gap Entrance Station, it is 16.1 miles to Fishers Gap Overlook.

TRAIL USE
Dayhiking, Backpacking

LENGTH
4.0 miles, 2–3 hours

CUMULATIVE ELEVATION +/-
-830'/+830'

DIFFICULTY
− 1 2 **3** 4 5 +

TRAIL TYPE
Loop

START & FINISH
N38° 32.008'
W78° 25.257'

FEATURES
Stream
Waterfalls
Wildflowers
Autumn Colors
Geologic Interest
Historic Interest

FACILITIES
None

Trail Description

Pick up the gated Rose River Fire Road on the east side of Skyline Drive. ▶1 Walk a few feet down Rose River Fire Road, and reach an intersection. The Skyland-Big Meadows Horse Trail crosses the fire road. Keep straight on Rose River Fire Road, descending along the gravel track in a hardwood forest dominated by maple and white oak. Small rills flow off Big Meadows above, then pass under the fire road via culvert. The track levels out among locust, land once farmed. Pass the Cave Cemetery on your right, atop a grassy hill at 0.5 mile. Watch for apple trees in this vicinity.

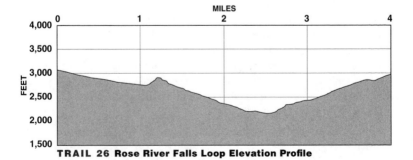
Historic Interest

Waterfall

Resume the descent. Hogcamp Branch falls loudly to your left. You soon walk along it. The forest canopy often opens along the roadbed, before reaching the junction with the Dark Hollow Falls Trail at a bridge over Hogcamp Branch at 1.0 mile. ▶2 Check out the 30-foot fall just above the bridge. A ribbon of frothing whitewater slices through a rock outcrop partially covered in moss. Turn right and head up the Dark Hollow Falls Trail. More falls tumble down as you head up, but you'll know Dark Hollow Falls. ▶3 It makes a wide drop, then gathers to tumble down three more tiers, a total descent of 70 feet. In summer the base of the falls is crowded,

TRAIL 26 Rose River Falls Loop Elevation Profile

Waterfall

since almost everyone has come from Skyline Drive on the Dark Hollow Falls Trail.

Return to Rose River Fire Road and cross the bridge. Just beyond here, the Rose River Loop Trail angles left and downhill along Hogcamp Branch. ▶4 Young hardwoods are replacing woolly adelgid–killed hemlocks and—for now—Dark Hollow is dark no more. Hogcamp Branch puts on a scenic display while stair-stepping down to meet the Rose River, falling and crashing in every type of fall, slide, cataract, and cascade, one tumbler after another, to gather in surprisingly deep pools, only to fall yet again. This is truly national park–level scenery. Black and yellow birch and maple comprise the hemlock-less forest. Note all the fallen hemlock trunks and limbs piled against streamside rocks. Hemlock is a soft wood and rots relatively quickly. At 2.0 miles, pass an open rock slab on the creek that lures hikers. A deep pool is at the base of the slab.

Stream

At 2.2 miles, reach a bridge spanning Hogcamp Branch. ▶5 The steel span arches well over and above Hogcamp Branch. The Rose River Loop then rock-hops a small stream. Reach the tailings of an old copper mine, with a path leading to the top of the tailings, back against a big bluff. Notice the stone and ironworks at the mine. This mine was opened in the early 1900s, but proved unprofitable and the shafts were filled. Keep downhill to reach a signpost near a large wooded flat. Turn left here and head upstream along the Rose River, which is crashing and dashing to your right, giving Hogcamp Branch a run for its scenic money.

Historic Interest

Stream

The Rose River Loop Trail leaves the river, climbing sharply in a fern forest, only to return at Rose River Falls at 2.8 miles. ▶6 Here, the water-course drops over a rock ledge about 25 feet, spreading out before reaching a pool. A spur trail leads downstream to a vista at lower Rose River Falls, which drops again as a narrow chute directly over a second ledge and out of sight from the viewing spot, making a splash in a large pool.

Beyond the falls, ascend a perched valley, under thriving hardwoods such as yellow birch and basswood. Reach another concrete signpost when meeting an old roadbed at 3.1 miles. Turn left here on a now wide trail, leaving the river. Rise into drier, oak-dominated woods to meet the Skyland-Big Meadows Horse Trail at 3.6 miles. ▶7 Stay left here, as the two trails run in conjunction, mostly climbing to reach the Rose River Fire Road. It is but a few steps to Skyline Drive from here. Complete your loop at 4.0 miles. ▶8

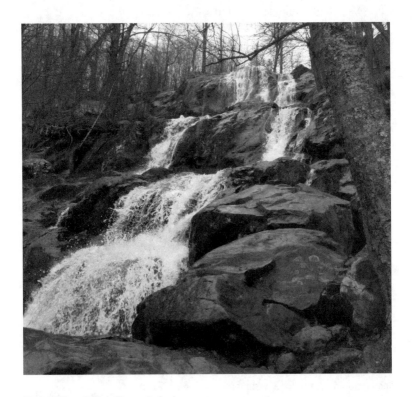

Dark Hollow Falls *spills over bedrock.*

⚐ MILESTONES

▶1 0.0 North end of Fishers Gap Overlook at milepost 49.4
▶2 1.0 Right on Dark Hollow Falls Trail
▶3 1.2 Dark Hollow Falls
▶4 1.4 Cross Hogcamp Branch, and left on Rose River Loop Trail
▶5 2.2 Bridge Hogcamp Branch
▶6 2.8 Rose River Falls
▶7 3.6 Stay left at Skyland-Big Meadows Horse Trail
▶8 4.0 North end of Fishers Gap Overlook at milepost 49.4

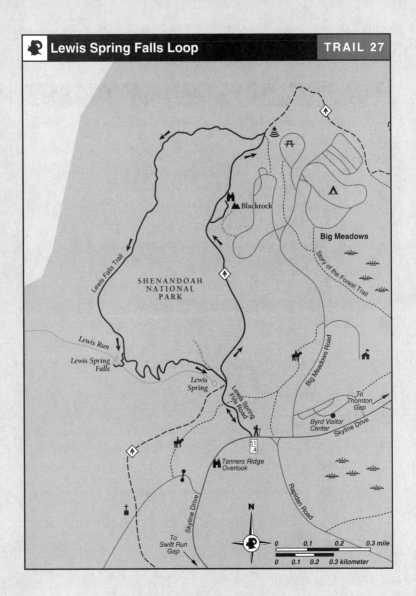

Blackrock

SHENANDOAH
NATIONAL
PARK

Lewis Falls Trail

Big Meadows

Story of the Forest Trail

Lewis Run

Lewis Spring
Falls

Lewis
Spring

Lewis Spring Fire Road

Big Meadows Road

Byrd Visitor
Center

To
Thornton
Gap

Skyline Drive

51
4

Tanners Ridge
Overlook

Skyline Drive

Rapidan Road

N

To
Swift Run
Gap

0   0.1   0.2   0.3 mile

0   0.1   0.2   0.3 kilometer

Lewis Spring Falls Loop

Don't forget the camera to capture the visual features along this hike that starts high and stays high. This loop takes place near the busy Big Meadows area, with its park lodge, visitor center, ranger station, and campground. Thus, this loop gets traffic, but deservedly so. Leave the parking area near Tanner Ridge Overlook, heading down Lewis Spring Service Road to reach the Appalachian Trail (AT). Walk northbound on the AT, climbing to Blackrock and its stellar views.

From there, the hike passes more interesting rock features, then joins the Lewis Falls Trail, where it descends to a loud, dramatic fall. Lewis Spring Falls is one of the highest elevation falls at Shenandoah. The distance is very doable, and the elevation changes aren't overly much, leaving you time to enjoy the other aspects of the greater Big Meadows area.

Best Time

In spring the falls rumble and the skies afford far-reaching views. Summer is good too, since this hike stays in the high country, but being near the main Big Meadows area can make it crowded. Fall can be busy too. Winter avails true solitude.

Finding the Trail

The parking area for the Lewis Spring Service Road is at milepost 51.4 on Skyline Drive. This parking area is sandwiched between the south entrance to Big Meadows and Tanners Ridge Overlook, on the west side of the road. The trailhead is 19.9 miles south of Thornton Gap Entrance Station.

TRAIL USE
Dayhiking

LENGTH
3.3 miles, 2–3 hours

CUMULATIVE ELEVATION +/-
+850'/-850'

DIFFICULTY
− 1 2 **3** 4 5 +

TRAIL TYPE
Loop

START & FINISH
N38° 31.020'
W78° 26.502'

FEATURES
Ridgeline
Stream
Summit
Waterfall
Autumn Colors
Wildflowers
Geologic Interest
Great Views

FACILITIES
Big Meadows Wayside
Visitor center
Campground
Lodge

Trail Description

This hike starts high
and stays high.

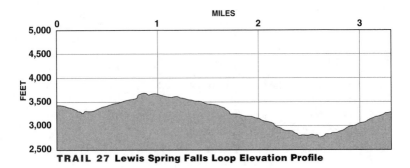

Autumn Colors

Ridgeline

Great Views

Summit

Leave the little parking area with several spots just
north of the Tanner Ridge Overlook. ►1 Walk a few
yards north along Skyline Drive to reach the Lewis
Spring Service Road. Pass around a chain gate,
then head downhill on a gravel track bordered by
a stunted high-country forest of haw, fire cherry,
and maple, reclaiming former fields. Look for apple,
birch, and locust trees too. The blue-blazed track
crosses the yellow-blazed Tanners Ridge Horse Trail
and continues descending.

At 0.2 mile, reach the Appalachian Trail (AT).
►2 Turn right here, heading northbound for Big
Meadows Lodge. Lewis Spring is immediately below
this intersection. Begin working uphill in hardwoods
mixed with pines, even a preserved hemlock or two.
Rocks and boulders of all sizes and descriptions are
strewn about the forest floor. The well-used path
features stonework to keep the trail from being
sloped. At 0.7 mile, reach a spur trail leading right
to Blackrock. ►3 Turn right here and make the 0.1-
mile climb to the outcrop, at 3,720 feet. ►4

Along the way, see if you can find a few red
spruce trees. In winter, they are easy to spot among
the barren hardwoods. Mountain ash clings to
the crags of Blackrock. The spiny rock protrusion
opens to the west, where you can see the towns

TRAIL 27 Lewis Spring Falls Loop Elevation Profile

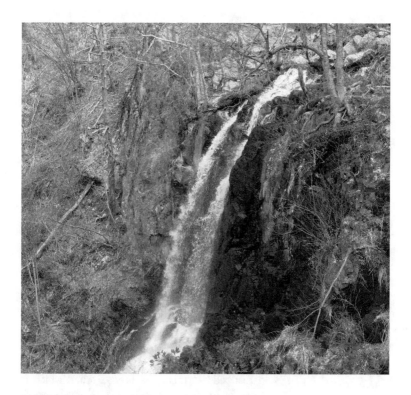

At high flows *Lewis Spring Falls shoots a white froth over a rock face.*

of Stanley and Luray in the Page Valley, amid the 180-degree view to the southwest and northwest, especially the high peaks of the park's north district. Below, the tops of oak trees seem close enough to touch. The AT can be seen below when the trees don't have leaves.

Return to the AT, curving below the rock massif of Blackrock. Another, smaller vista lies off the trail. Ahead, pass below the Big Meadows Lodge before meeting the Lewis Spring Falls Trail at 1.3 miles. ▶5 Here, turn acutely left on the Lewis Spring Falls Trail amid lush woods with a ferny understory. Continue downslope, looking for a level grassy spot

 Wildflowers

near the trail good for picnicking, at 1.6 miles. Keep south along the western escarpment of the mountain, which drops off to your right. At 1.9 miles, the trail skirts below a lichen-covered rock protrusion.

Geologic Interest

Beyond here, the rocky trail steepens beneath the woods. Curve onto a southwest-facing slope, with mountain laurel and pines joining the sturdy oaks. Outcrops along the trail provide views into the hollow of upper Hawksbill Creek, which becomes audible. Reach another junction at 2.5 miles. ►6 Here, a spur trail leads right to an outcrop and

Great Views

view into the valley below and lands beyond. Massanutten Mountain forms a backdrop. The main spur path crosses wide and rocky Hawksbill Creek

Stream

and then curves beyond a precipice. A guardrail guides you the last bit to a rock-walled observation

Waterfall

point. ►7 Here, you can look down at the 81-foot falls spilling over the rock face crashing into rocks and then splashing out of sight.

Backtrack to the Lewis Falls Trail, and begin a switchback-filled ascent along Hawksbill Creek, ►8 drifting into rich waterside woods and drier pine-oak forest away from the stream. Join an old roadbed, ►9 then pass Lewis Spring, which is housed in a rock-and-wood structure with a visible outflow. Just ahead, reach the AT again, at 3.1 miles. To your right is another boxed spring, and the site of the long dismantled Lewis Spring Shelter. From here, keep straight on the gravel road, backtracking to the trailhead. ►10

🚶 MILESTONES

▶1   0.0   Lewis Spring Service Road parking area at milepost 51.4

▶2   0.2   Right, northbound, on the AT

▶3   0.7   Spur to Blackrock

▶4   0.8   Vista from Blackrock

▶5   1.3   Acute left on Lewis Spring Falls Trail

▶6   2.5   Spur to vista and Lewis Spring Falls observation platform

▶7   2.6   Lewis Spring Falls observation platform and backtrack

▶8   2.7   Ascend along Hawksbill Creek

▶9   3.1   Complete loop at AT, and backtrack on Lewis Spring
          Service Road

▶10 3.3   Return to parking area

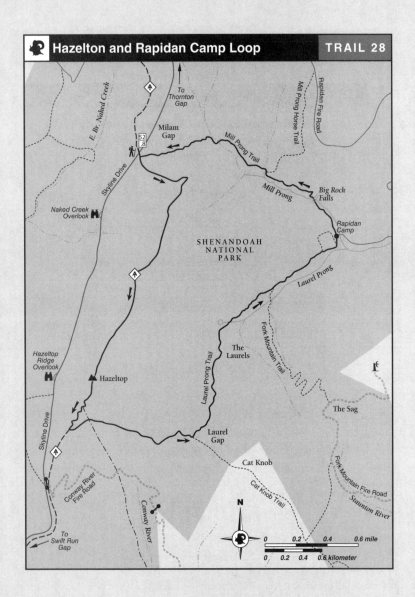

To Thornton Gap

E. Br. Naked Creek

Milam Gap

Mill Prong Trail

Mill Prong Horse Trail

Rapidan Fire Road

52
8

Skyline Drive

Naked Creek Overlook

Mill Prong

Big Rock Falls

Rapidan Camp

SHENANDOAH NATIONAL PARK

Laurel Prong

Hazeltop Ridge Overlook

Hazeltop

Laurel Prong Trail

The Laurels

Fork Mountain Trail

The Sag

Skyline Drive

Laurel Gap

Cat Knob

Cat Knob Trail

Fork Mountain Fire Road

Staunton River

Conway River Fire Road

Conway River

N

To Swift Run Gap

0   0.2   0.4   0.6 mile

0   0.2   0.4   0.6 kilometer

Hazeltop and Rapidan Camp Loop

This loop takes you over Hazeltop, the third highest peak in the park, and then traces attractive Laurel Prong Trail down to Rapidan Camp, the woodland getaway of President Herbert Hoover (1929–33). There's much to see at the camp; you can even embark on a self-guided interpretive tour. Return to Milam Gap via Mill Prong Trail, and view Big Rock Falls along the way.

Best Time

This is a good summertime destination. The hike is shaded in greenery then, and you can see historic Rapidan Camp at the time of year when President Herbert Hoover used it to escape the brutal summers in Washington, D.C.

Finding the Trail

The Milam Gap Trailhead is located at milepost 52.8, on the west side of Skyline Drive. It can be reached by driving north on Skyline Drive for 12.7 miles from the Swift Run Gap Entrance Station. The Appalachian Trail (AT) is accessible behind the parking area. Start your hike here.

Trail Description

Head southbound on the AT from the Milam Gap parking area. ▶1 Note the preponderance of apple trees in this area. Bears gorge on them in fall. Cross Skyline Drive and come to a trail junction. To your left is Mill Prong Trail, your return route. Continue

TRAIL USE
Dayhiking, Backpacking
LENGTH
7.2 miles, 6 hours
(includes 1 hour at
Rapidan Camp)
**CUMULATIVE
ELEVATION +/-**
+1,300'/-1,300'
DIFFICULTY
− 1 2 3 **4** 5 +
TRAIL TYPE
Loop
START & FINISH
N38° 30.013'
W78° 26.759'

FEATURES
Stream
Ridgeline
Summit
Waterfall
Great Views
Autumn Colors
Wildlife
Wildflowers
Historic Interest

FACILITIES
None

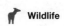 **Wildlife**

▲ Ridgeline

🔭 Great Views

👤 Summit

gently uphill, southbound on the AT through a forest shading fields of ferns, and reach a sharp right turn at mile 0.4. Now you are really going south as the AT heads toward Hazeltop.

The trail grade is nearly level, but it rises slightly on a slowly narrowing ridge. At points the AT is arrow straight. Note the trailside upthrust rocks. At 1.9 miles, a spur leads right to a rocky overlook. ▶2 Here, you can enjoy an open view to the west, of the South Fork Shenandoah River Valley and waves of mountains in the distance. Achieve the peak of Hazeltop (3,812 feet) at 2.0 miles. To your right is a gnarled oak next to a large embedded rock, the actual summit. To the left of the trail is a small balsam fir, a survivor of the forests that now thrive much farther north in New England and Canada. Its needles are flat, fragrant, and friendly (not sharp). Leave the summit, and come to a left turn. To your right are two red spruce trees, another member of the Canadian forest. Its needles are a darker green, rounded, and sharp. These trees grow in only a few locations in the park.

The AT drops moderately and approaches the scenic Laurel Prong Trail at mile 2.4. ▶3 Turn left on Laurel Prong Trail. Several springs flow over the boulder-laden slope. The going is slow on the irregular tread. The Conway River Valley falls away

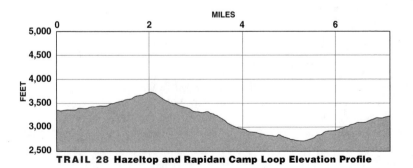

TRAIL 28 Hazeltop and Rapidan Camp Loop Elevation Profile

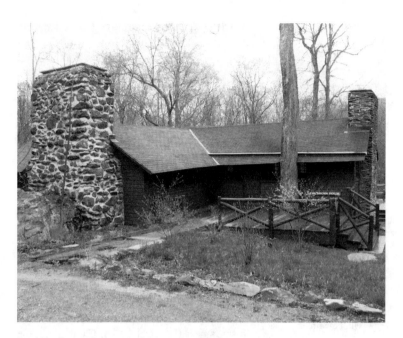

Rapidan Camp, *Herbert Hoover's presidential backcountry retreat*

to your right. The trail descends sharply, levels off, and then makes a final dip to arrive at Laurel Gap and a trail junction at 3.4 miles. ▶4 Cat Knob looms to the east. This is a good place to take a break—if the winds aren't howling.

Turn left, staying on the Laurel Prong Trail. It continues to drop sharply while snaking through "The Laurels," a concentration of mountain laurel and likely the inspiration for the stream's name. Backpackers find legal campsites along this section of trail, but remember, you can't camp within a half mile of Rapidan Camp. Pass a spring at 3.9 miles, the first of several rills flowing off Hazeltop. A few hemlock trees are hanging on. The valley forest is in transition. Rock-hop Laurel Prong at 4.1 miles. Watch for stone fences from pioneer farming days. At 4.7 miles, Fork Mountain Trail leaves right, ▶5

Visit one of America's first presidential retreats.

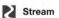 **Stream**

into a thicket of rhododendron that is perhaps yet another inspiration for the stream's name; mountaineers often called rhododendron "laurel" and mountain laurel "ivy." Confusing, huh?

Continue straight on the Laurel Prong Trail. A spur trail leads left to Five Tents, the original dwelling site for Herbert Hoover. When the president first came here, workmen built five tents on platforms, around which a cabin was ultimately constructed. You can still see the fireplace. Arrive at Rapidan Camp at 5.3 miles. ▶6 Situated at the confluence of Laurel Prong and Mill Creek, the camp lies in a lovely wooded setting. Walk around, and check out the three buildings and interpretive information. There are short nature trails here too. This place is engaging, so give it at least an hour. Imagine the president and his compadres strategizing on subjects of national import—trout fishing too. Back then hemlocks shaded and cooled the flat.

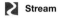 **Historic Interest**

 Wildflowers

Stream

Waterfall

Continue your loop hike on the Mill Prong Trail, which starts near the Creel Cabin. Climb along the steep valley, rife with wildflowers in spring. The trail now drops to Mill Prong, crossing it below Big Rock Falls at mile 5.7. ▶7 Big Rock Falls slips 15 feet over a rock slide into a large, deep pool. President Hoover surely slung a fly rod here.

The trail switchbacks, levels off in a rocky section, and intersects the Mill Prong Horse Trail at mile 6.1. ▶8 Bear left, still on the Mill Prong Trail, crossing a side branch, and then rock-hop Mill Prong once more at 6.6 miles. ▶9 The stream is now wide, shallow, and pocked with stones. The path leads into an open, ferny forest. Enter a grassy glade before intersecting the AT at mile 7.2. ▶10 Turn right on the AT, cross Skyline Drive, and return to the Milam Gap Trailhead.

🚶 MILESTONES

►1　0.0　Milam Gap parking area at milepost 52.8

►2　1.9　Spur leaves right to overlook on Hazeltop

►3　2.4　Left on Laurel Prong Trail

►4　3.4　Left at Laurel Gap, still on Laurel Prong Trail

►5　4.7　Fork Mountain Trail leaves right

►6　5.3　Rapidan Camp

►7　5.7　Big Rock Falls

►8　6.1　Mill Prong Horse Trail leaves right

►9　6.6　Cross Mill Prong

►10　7.2　Meet AT, and return to parking area

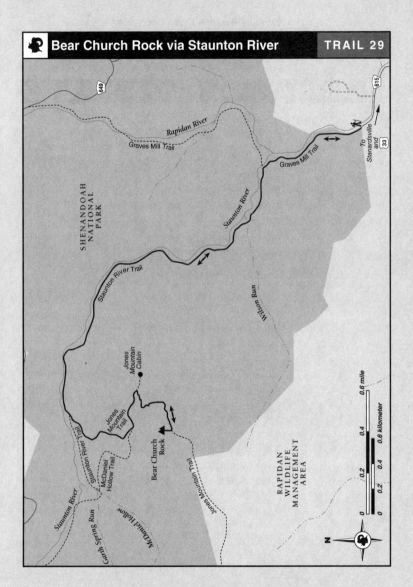

Bear Church Rock via Staunton River

Bear Church Rock is one of the all-time top names in Appalachia. The origin is lost to time, but from the granite outcrop it doesn't take much imagination to visualize a pulpit overlooking the Staunton River Valley. The pulpit lies below the main granite crag where your views open. Conjuring up a bear preaching a sermon may prove more difficult, but some claim the panorama to be a near-religious experience. Your hike to the crag is rewarding too. The Staunton River tumbles in pools and cascades impressive for the limited stream volume. Be apprised that the nearly 2,000-foot elevation change is challenging.

Best Time

This hike is great year-round. The low-elevation trailhead makes it accessible in winter. You can enjoy streamside scenery without having to ford any streams. The Staunton River Valley presents wildflowers and cascades in spring and summer, while great views can be had from Bear Church Rock in autumn.

Finding the Trail

From US 33 Business in Stanardsville, east of Swift Run Gap, take VA 230, Madison Road, north for 7.1 miles to VA 662. Turn left on VA 662, Graves Mill Road. Follow VA 662 for 5.1 miles, then turn right onto Graves Road, which is still VA 662 (the road going forward here becomes VA 615). Immediately bridge Kinsey Run, and follow Graves Road to dead-end at the Graves Mill Trailhead at 1.2 miles.

TRAIL USE
Dayhiking, Backpacking

LENGTH
7.6 miles, 4½–5½ hours

CUMULATIVE ELEVATION +/-
+1,950'/-1,950'

DIFFICULTY
− 1 2 3 4 **5** +

TRAIL TYPE
Out & Back

START & FINISH
N38° 26.219'
W78° 22.003'

FEATURES
Stream
Ridgeline
Waterfall
Wildflowers
Autumn Colors
Great Views
Secluded
Geologic Interest
Swimming

FACILITIES
None

Trail Description

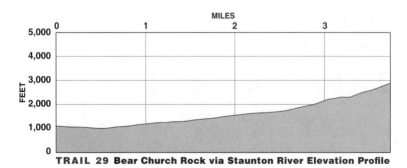

Leave the VA 615 trailhead on the Graves Mill Trail, passing around vehicle barrier boulders. ▶1 The Rapidan River rushes to your right. This is a popular fishing area, and you may see anglers along the many pools on the river. Make an easy trek up a nearly level valley, under towering hardwoods dominated by black birch, sycamore, and beech, with an odd cedar thrown in. Ferns are scattered across the forest floor.

At 0.5 mile, join the Staunton River Trail. ▶2 The Staunton River, a major mountain tributary of the Rapidan River, forms east of the Blue Ridge below Fork Mountain. By this point it is a full-fledged mountain cataract with alternating rapids and pools. The trail gradient increases, and you soon come alongside the Staunton River just in time to view a 15-foot slide cascade spilling over a rock slab. You can reach it on a short spur trail.

The Staunton River Trail continues up the wide, sloped valley, once cultivated by mountaineers, but now growing spring wildflowers under cucumber magnolias and tulip trees. Rock piles are especially visible when the leaves are off. Step over possibly dry Wilson Run at 0.9 mile. Continue up the valley in tight but spindly tree stands broken up by larger, more robust woods. At 1.3 miles, bisect a pair of huge boulder gates. ▶3 Leap rocky overflow braids

Stream

Autumn Colors

Swimming

Waterfall

Wildflowers

TRAIL 29 Bear Church Rock via Staunton River Elevation Profile

MILES

FEET

from the Staunton River as well as rivulets flowing off Jones Mountain above you. Yellow birches appear as the path gains elevation. At 1.8 miles, watch for the foundations of an old homesite on your left, with many rock piles and stone fences as well.

At 2.6 miles, the hike veers left onto the Jones Mountain Trail. ►4 The ascent escalates, and watery sounds fade along the boulder-strewn hillside. Intersect the McDaniel Hollow Trail at 3.0 miles, following a short but steep burst. ►5 Stay left with the Jones Mountain Trail, curving through tunnels of mountain laurel. The path levels off and then meets the Jones Mountain Cabin spur trail at 3.3 miles. ►6 The dwelling, once home to pre-park resident Harvey Nichols, is available for overnight rental. It is maintained by the Potomac Appalachian Trail Club. For rental information visit **www.patc.net.**

Resume climbing toward Bear Church Rock, switchbacking up the east end of Jones Mountain. Reach a trail split at the crest of Jones Mountain. Turn right here and emerge onto multiple granite outcrops, broken by windswept trees clinging to crevices. ►7 The escarpment exposes the park's glory. Fork Mountain, Doubletop Mountain, and the crest of the Blue Ridge stand out. The rocky cone of Old Rag peeks above nearby ridges. Below, Staunton River and its tributaries carve a wooded valley. Both bears and humans are rewarded on Bear Church Rock.

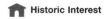 **Historic Interest**

 Steep

Bear Church Rock is a difficult and remote destination.

▲ **Ridgeline**

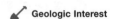 **Geologic Interest**

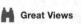 **Great Views**

🚶	**MILESTONES**	
►1	0.0	Graves Mill Trailhead
►2	0.5	Right on Staunton River Trail
►3	1.3	Boulder gates
►4	2.6	Left on Jones Mountain Trail
►5	3.0	McDaniel Hollow Trail leaves right
►6	3.3	Spur to Jones Mountain Cabin
►7	3.8	Bear Church Rock

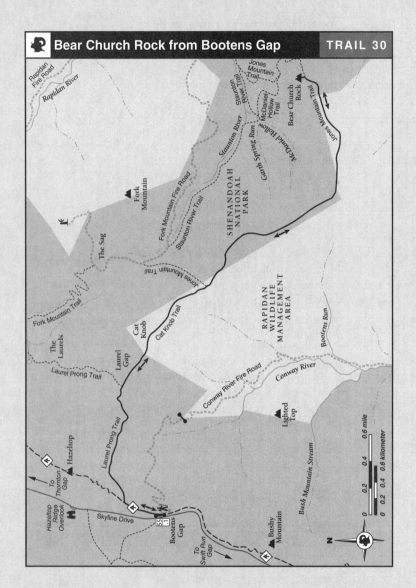

Bear Church Rock from Bootens Gap

This solitude-laden high-country hike leads along the ridge of Jones Mountain to an incredible view from Bear Church Rock. The hiking along Jones Mountain is some of Shenandoah's finest. You are above 3,000 feet most of the hike, yet the trail is never steep for long and is level much of the way, making it about the easiest 9 mountain miles you can ask for. The whole hike is on hiker-only foot trails, meandering through varied and beautiful forests. It is a great way to spend a day in Shenandoah. Make sure to bring water.

Best Time

This hike is great during all seasons. You can experience clear views in fall, winter, and spring, while summer avails cool temperatures. Solitude can be found any time.

Finding the Trail

Bootens Gap is located at milepost 55.1 on Skyline Drive. From the Swift Run Gap Entrance Station, head north on Skyline Drive for 10.4 miles to the Bootens Gap parking area. The small parking area will be on your right, the east side of Skyline Drive. Pick up the Appalachian Trail (AT) here.

Trail Description

Walk just a few steps down Conway Fire Road, ▶1 then reach the AT. Turn left, northbound, as the AT ascends moderately up the southwest side of

TRAIL USE
Dayhiking

LENGTH
9.4 miles, 5–6½ hours

CUMULATIVE ELEVATION +/-
-800'/+800'

DIFFICULTY
– 1 2 3 **4** 5 +

TRAIL TYPE
Out & Back

START & FINISH
N38° 28.106'
W78° 27.446'

FEATURES
Ridgeline
Autumn Colors
Geologic Interest
Great Views
Secluded

FACILITIES
None

Stay above 3,000 feet nearly the entire hike.

Geologic Interest

Ridgeline

Autumn Colors

Hazeltop, coming to a trail junction at 0.4 mile. ►2 Turn right on the Laurel Prong Trail. The footbed descends past several springs on a boulder-laden slope, flowing from Hazeltop. The trail drops sharply just before arriving at breezy Laurel Gap and another trail junction at 1.4 miles. ►3 Keep straight, joining the short Cat Knob Trail. Follow the faint footbed uphill, twisting and turning among impressive gray boulders. Enter a slice of the Rapidan Wildlife Management Area at mile 1.8.

The trail makes one last jump and then descends slightly before intersecting the Jones Mountain Trail at 2.1 miles. ►4 It has come up 0.8 mile from The Sag, a simple but memorable Appalachian landmark name. Veer right, now on the Jones Mountain Trail.

The ridge-running path makes for pleasant walking among windswept oaks. The fern and grass understory, mingled with mountain laurel, adds more appeal. A sense of seclusion overwhelms the ridgeline. The little-used trail descends, making an unexpected right at mile 2.4. Come to a gap in a broken forest. The brush may crowd the path in late summer. Reenter the park at mile 2.7 in oak woodland. Begin an extensive, level stretch, trending slightly downhill. The scenery is among Shenandoah's finest.

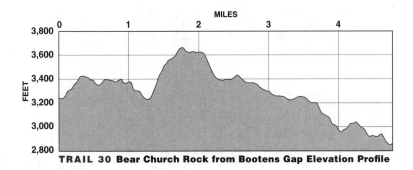

TRAIL 30 Bear Church Rock from Bootens Gap Elevation Profile

In a grassy gap at mile 3.6, the trail turns left and down, east toward Bear Church Rock and away from Bluff Mountain. ▶5 Look for an outcrop on your left with warm-up views of Fork Mountain. Begin a more-down-than-not roller-coaster ride along Jones Mountain. Large granite outcrops rise among the hardwoods.

At mile 4.6, the trail zigzags very steeply down the point of the ridge among brush and laurel. Watch for a side trail splitting left in 0.1 mile. This side trail emerges onto the granite slab of Bear Church Rock. ▶6 The sloping rock creates a natural viewing platform. Look for water-filled potholes in the near and mountains aplenty in the far. What a perch!

 Great Views

From here, you can see Fork Mountain, Doubletop Mountain, and the crest of the Blue Ridge. The Staunton River Valley cuts a chasm below. This is one of my favorite overlooks in the entire park, and I have never seen a soul while up here. Explore the various outcrops broken by screens of vegetation, as well as at the base of the outcrops. Make sure to allow plenty of time to return.

 Secluded

MILESTONES

▶1	0.0	Bootens Gap parking area at milepost 55.1
▶2	0.4	Right on Laurel Prong Trail
▶3	1.4	Join Cat Knob Trail
▶4	2.1	Pick up Jones Mountain Trail
▶5	3.6	Turn left, away from Bluff Mountain
▶6	4.7	Bear Church Rock

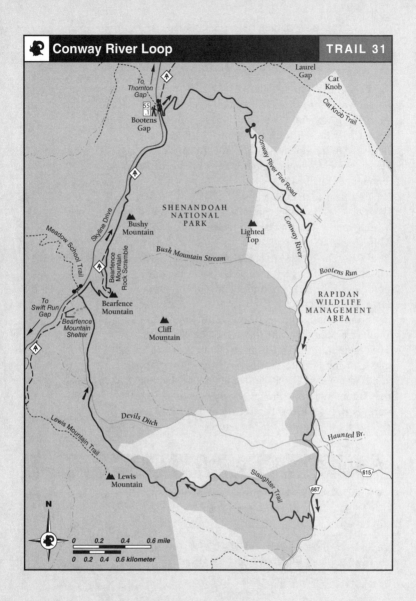

Conway River Loop

TRAIL 31

Laurel
Gap

Cat
Knob

Cat Knob Trail

To
Thornton
Gap

55
1

Bootens
Gap

Conway River Fire Road

Conway River

SHENANDOAH
NATIONAL
PARK

Bushy
Mountain

Lighted
Top

Meadow School Trail

Skyline Drive

Bush Mountain Stream

Bootens Run

Bearfence Mountain Rock Scramble

RAPIDAN
WILDLIFE
MANAGEMENT
AREA

To
Swift Run
Gap

Bearfence
Mountain

Bearfence
Mountain
Shelter

Cliff
Mountain

Lewis Mountain Trail

Devils Ditch

Haunted Br.

615

Lewis
Mountain

Slaughter Trail

667

N

0   0.2   0.4   0.6 mile

0   0.2   0.4   0.6 kilometer

Conway River Loop

This loop leaves the Blue Ridge and follows the scenic Conway River through a parcel of the Rapidan Wildlife Management Area. Leave the Conway River, and head into the high country on the seldom trampled Slaughter Trail, passing a pioneer homesite, for the upper reaches of Devils Ditch. Complete your trip by clambering over Bearfence Mountain, with its 360-degree views, on a short but challenging rock and boulder scramble; *pets are prohibited on this scramble.* This loop makes for a long dayhike but a great one- or even two-night backpack.

Take note that Rapidan Wildlife Management Area, managed by the State of Virginia, has hunting as well as different camping rules from Shenandoah National Park. Please consult the latest information at Virginia Department of Game and Inland Fisheries website (**www.dgif.virginia.gov**).

Best Time

This challenging loop has it all: views, waterfalls, streams, and ridges—something for every season. Spring has extensive vistas, wildflowers, and bold streams. But it is double-edged since the hike requires three fords of the Conway River. Summer is cool on the river, and fall presents colors and even lower water. The views from atop Bearfence Mountain are great after the first cold fronts move through. Winter can be tough with the stream crossings.

TRAIL USE
Dayhiking,
Backpacking,
Pets Prohibited

LENGTH
12.0 miles, 7–9 hours

**CUMULATIVE
ELEVATION +/-**
-2,300'/+2,300'

DIFFICULTY
– 1 2 3 4 **5** +

TRAIL TYPE
Loop

START & FINISH
N38° 28.106'
W78° 27.446'

FEATURES
Ridgeline
Stream
Waterfall
Wildflowers
Old-Growth
Autumn Colors
Geologic Interest
Historic Interest
Great Views

FACILITIES
None

Finding the Trail

This highlight offers attractions for every season.

The Conway River Fire Road starts at Bootens Gap at milepost 55.1 on Skyline Drive. From the Swift Run Gap Entrance Station, head north on Skyline Drive for 10.4 miles to the Bootens Gap parking area. The small parking area will be on your right on the east side of Skyline Drive. Conway River Fire Road starts in the back of the parking area.

Trail Description

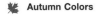 **Autumn Colors**

Leave the Bootens Gap parking area on Conway River Fire Road. ▶1 The wide, grassy track makes two switchbacks before coming to the upper Conway River. It may be dry here in fall. Dive deeper into the valley, where bigger hardwoods trees rise.

Pass through a gate at 1.4 miles, and enter the Rapidan Wildlife Management Area (Rapidan WMA). ▶2 Red blazes mark the boundary between the national park and the wildlife area. Swing back left and cross an often-dry ravine at mile 1.6. Over the next couple of miles you may see a 4WD vehicle on the track. Rough 4WD roads splinter off the main path. Step over a fair-sized stream at mile 2.2, then come to another decent-sized but unnamed stream at 2.6 miles. ▶3 A 25-foot

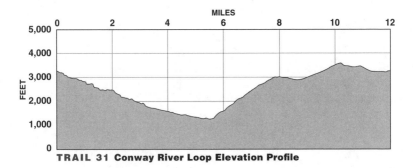

TRAIL 31 Conway River Loop Elevation Profile

Waterfall

wet weather fall tumbles in stages about 40 yards upstream from the trail (roadbed) you are on. Follow this tributary downstream.

Arrive at a fork in the road at 2.8 miles. The left fork leads to a large clearing. Stay on the right fork, leading to Bootens Run at 3.3 miles. Rock-hop Bootens Run, then come alongside the boulder-strewn Conway River. The trout-filled, boulder-laden, large watercourse presents everywhere-you-look beauty. The national park is on the far side of the stream.

Stream

At 3.8 miles, come to a concrete Shenandoah National Park trail signpost. ▶4 Here, VA 615 leads left. Stay right on the Conway River Trail, and shortly come to your first crossing of the Conway River. It should be a simple rock-hop in summer and fall, but can be a ford in winter and spring. Make your way carefully across the river, leaving any potential jeep traffic behind.

Wildflowers

The Conway River, with its deep pools for fishing or wading, is now on your left. Travel a riverside rocky track under dense forest. At 4.4 miles, reach a wide flat with rock piles, indicating former farmland. Rock-hop Devils Ditch at mile 4.8. ▶5 As with most Shenandoah streams, flow can range from a trickle to a torrent. Pass a Rapidan WMA hunting trail that leads right, up the Devils Ditch.

Come to another ford of the Conway River at mile 5.0. ▶6 Big boulders and deep water make this ford tough during high water. Evidence of flood damage can be seen along the river—piled tree trunks, scoured roots, and jumbled rocks. The

Stream

trail leads uphill under scads of white pines, then descends back to the Conway. Come to your third and final river crossing at 5.5 miles. ▶7 This deep pool is a great summertime swimming hole. Cross the river here; this ford will likely get you wet, yet it's easier than the one just upstream. VA 667 is just 0.3 mile down a jeep road after the river crossing.

Come to the concrete signpost for the Slaughter Trail, and begin heading upstream. You will be in Shenandoah National Park the remainder of the hike. The Conway River should now be on your right. The rocky Slaughter Trail briefly parallels the Conway. Look for the rock walls and exotic bushes of an old riverside homesite. The Slaughter Trail leaves the river, climbing steeply up a spur ridge leading toward Lewis Mountain. Notice the old-growth white pines above you.

Historic Interest

Old-Growth

The path switchbacks left at mile 5.7 and then steepens even more before leveling off at mile 6.5. Congratulations, you have just climbed 850 feet in 1 mile. Traverse a gap, pass a rock pile, climb a little more, and then come to a homesite on your right. The chimney and foundation are crumbling. A spring is on the far side of the homesite. You might

Crossing a view-laden perch *along Bearfence Mountain Rock Scramble*

If you want to do the Bearfence Mountain Rock Scramble, it can be accessed from milepost 56.4 on Skyline Drive. The scramble is only a 1.2-mile loop from the parking lot; however, allow ample time and bring your camera on a clear day.

want to rest and explore the homesite because more climbing lies ahead.

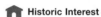 **Historic Interest**

Keep ascending on the eroded trail, passing blazed boundary trees. Pass the ruins of an out-building on your left and a split-rail fence on your right. At mile 7.3 beneath a yellow birch, a rock-lined spring sends forth cool water. The moss- and grass-covered trail nears Lewis Mountain and levels out at mile 7.7. Watch as an old road leaves left for the crest of Lewis Mountain. Cruise along the east slope of the mountain, earning a little rest after climbing 1,750 feet since the Conway River.

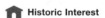 **Historic Interest**

Start an irregular descent to jump the upper Devils Ditch at 8.6 miles. ►8 Mountain laurel shades the valley of upper Devils Ditch. The grassy trail is easy on your feet and lungs. Parallel the upper Devils Ditch to a road fork at 9.4 miles. Here, a roadbed leaves left to the Bearfence Mountain Shelter. Keep straight and meet the Appalachian Trail (AT) at 9.5 miles. ►9 Turn right, northbound.

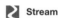 **Stream**

Ascend the AT through intertwined mountain laurel and squatty pines, gaining the southwest side of Bearfence Mountain. Switchback uphill among lichen-covered boulders, passing a rock on your right that has views of Bluff Mountain to the east. Come to Bearfence Mountain Loop Trail at 10.1 miles. ►10 Turn right, taking the loop trail, and keep climbing. A short trail leads left to the obscure crest of Bearfence Mountain. Descend a bit and pass an outcrop on your left at 10.2 miles. ►11 It offers spectacular views of Skyline Drive, Massanutten Mountain, and the Shenandoah Valley below.

 Great Views

Come to the Bearfence Mountain Rock Scramble, marked with a concrete signpost, and turn right. The scramble is doable with a full backpack, *but it is closed to pets.* Carefully follow the blue blazes. Fantastic panoramas open in all directions, including the Conway River drainage from where you came. Fork Mountain, Jones Mountain, and Cat Knob rise across the Conway. This is one of the best views in the park. Continue scrambling amid upthrust rocks with more views. Return to the AT at mile 10.6, and turn right. ►12 It feels like a walk in the park. Skirt the edge of Bush Mountain beneath some large oak trees. A prolonged descent nears Skyline Drive. Slip over to the northeast side of the Blue Ridge. Wildflowers are abundant in spring here, from trillium to jack-in-the-pulpit. Reach Conway River Fire Road at mile 12.0. Take a few steps left on the fire road, and complete your loop. ►13

Great Views

Geologic Interest

▲ **Ridgeline**

Wildflowers

MILESTONES

►1	0.0	Bootens Gap parking area at milepost 55.1
►2	1.4	Gate into Rapidan Wildlife Management Area
►3	2.6	Waterfall about 40 yards up a side stream
►4	3.8	Cross Conway River
►5	4.8	Cross Devils Ditch
►6	5.0	Cross Conway River
►7	5.5	Cross Conway River, and pick up Slaughter Trail
►8	8.6	Cross upper Devils Ditch
►9	9.5	Right on AT
►10	10.1	Right on Bearfence Mountain Loop Trail
►11	10.2	Enjoy view and then right at Bearfence Mountain Rock Scramble
►12	10.6	Right on AT
►13	12.0	Complete loop

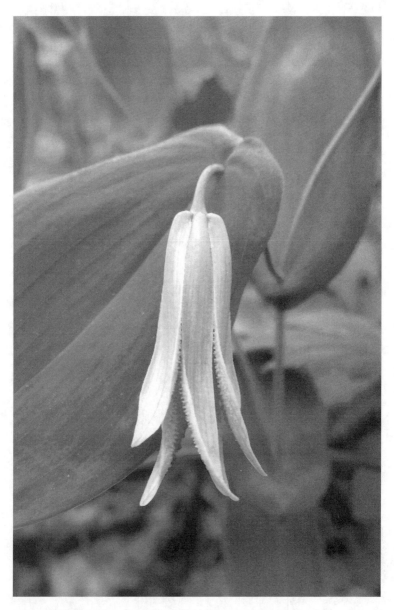

Mountain bellwort *graces the Conway River Valley.*

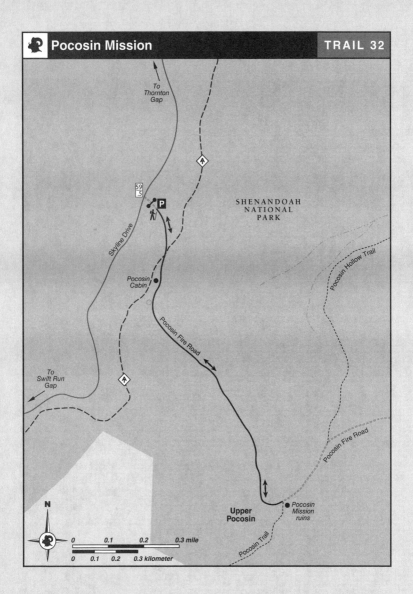

Pocosin Mission

TRAIL 32

To
Thornton
Gap

SHENANDOAH
NATIONAL
PARK

59
5

P

Skyline Drive

Pocosin Hollow Trail

Pocosin
Cabin

Pocosin Fire Road

To
Swift Run
Gap

Pocosin Fire Road

N

0   0.1   0.2   0.3 mile

0   0.1   0.2   0.3 kilometer

**Upper
Pocosin**

Pocosin
Mission
ruins

Pocosin Trail

Pocosin Mission

Take a walk into the past on this short trek. Leave Skyline Drive on the wide and easy Pocosin Fire Road, and explore the ruins of the Pocosin Mission, where a brave Episcopal minister attempted to save the souls of surrounding mountaineers. Explore the ruins of the mission and other nearby signs of habitation on a child-friendly walk. If you desire to walk a bit more, you can head down Pocosin Hollow. Descend to see many old-growth trees on your way down to a tumbling watercourse, where you'll find a nice spot to picnic or relax. Or you can take a stroll on an adjacent parcel of the Appalachian Trail (AT), and grab a view from a rocky slope.

Best Time

Since the hike is short, you can enjoy it any time of year. However, in spring you can view wildflowers and also better view the relics of the Pocosin Mission.

Finding the Trail

From Swift Run Gap, drive north on Skyline Drive for 6 miles to milepost 59.5. Look on your right for a road and a sign saying "Do Not Block Fire Road." Turn onto this road, and park in one of the gravel spots. The Pocosin Fire Road starts here. This road is 0.4 mile south of The Oaks Overlook and 1.6 miles north of Bald Face Mountain Overlook.

TRAIL USE
Dayhiking,
Child-Friendly

LENGTH
2.0 miles, 1–2 hours

**CUMULATIVE
ELEVATION +/-**
-420'/+420'

DIFFICULTY
– 1 **2** 3 4 5 +

TRAIL TYPE
Out & Back

START & FINISH
N38° 24.798'
W78° 29.318'

FEATURES
Ridgeline
Wildflowers
Autumn Colors
Old-Growth
Historic Interest
Great Views

FACILITIES
None

Trail Description

It's a short walk
to these historic
mission ruins.

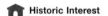 **Autumn Colors**

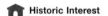 **Historic Interest**

A lot of hikers miss this trailhead since it has a narrow entrance. After you find it, leave the parking area on the Pocosin Fire Road, a nearly level wide grade. ▶1 Intersect the AT at 0.1 mile. ▶2 A northern hardwood forest of red maple, sugar maple, basswood, and cherry rise overhead. Distinguishing between sugar maples and red maples is easy. Look at the leaf of a sugar maple. The curves between lobes of the sugar maple are "U" shaped, whereas the curves between lobes of the red maple are at right angles. Continue on the Pocosin Fire Road and come to a clearing at 0.2 mile. ▶3 This is the Pocosin Cabin, built in 1937 by the Civilian Conservation Corps. The Potomac Appalachian Trail Club (PATC), a philanthropic organization that maintains trails, rents this cabin to its members.

The fire road drops moderately, still bordered by deciduous trees. The trail's width makes for easy hiking, and you soon pass a spring on trail left. It is used by AT hikers and those staying at the cabin. Come to a trail junction at 1.0 mile. ▶4 This spot is known as Upper Pocosin. To your right, through the trees, are the remnants of the Pocosin Mission.

Follow the footpath to the steps of the old church, built in 1904. Look at the walls made of native stone. The other nearby building is barely

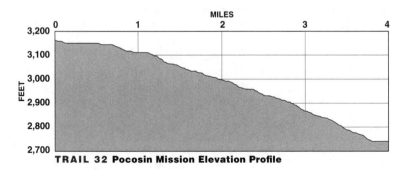

TRAIL 32 Pocosin Mission Elevation Profile

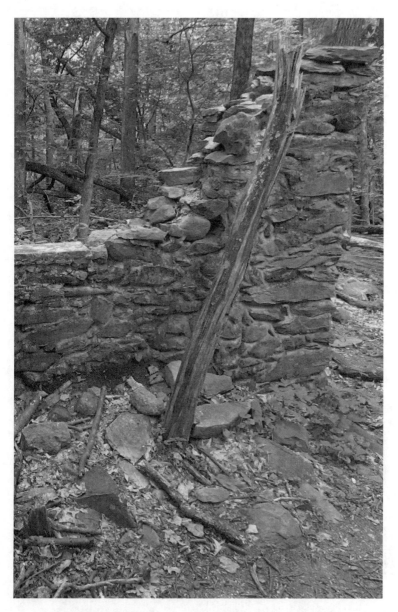

Stone foundations *of the Pocosin Mission stand silent in Shenandoah's highland woods.*

About Old-Growth Forests

FLORA

Sometimes an old-growth forest isn't as evident as people expect. Before you imagine a continuous stand of giant trees, you must realize that an authentic old-growth woodland is not an agglomeration of evenly aged trees. On the contrary, a forest made up of evenly aged trees is a sign of disturbance. An old-growth forest will have many big trees along with younger trees that grow when they get the chance. When a big tree falls, it creates a light gap. Young trees sprout in this light gap, and other already somewhat grown trees thrive in the additional sun. Trees are continually growing and dying, as older trees succumb to lightning strikes, disease, or old age, creating a mosaic of trees of all ages.

standing. Parts of the structure were built with hand-hewn logs; boards, nails, and even tar paper were later additions. Watch below you, as there is much broken glass, some parcels of clay pipe, and even pottery shards around. Look around also for the cemetery, where a few graves are marked with simple stones. As you tour the area, imagine the work of these missionaries, here in the remote Potomac Highlands, trying to spread Christianity among folk who had rarely traveled more than a day's horseback ride from home.

If you are looking for more trail mileage, head for Pocosin Hollow. To get there, continue down the Pocosin Fire Road, and veer left on the Pocosin Hollow Trail in a quarter mile. From this point forward, you should have the nut- and acorn-lined trail to yourself. Look for large old-growth trees scattered here and there along the path. The hike passes a boulder field before entering a wet draw, a rich wildflower area. Numerous old-growth yellow birch, oak, and tulip trees rise overhead. Reach the main watercourse of Pocosin Hollow, a tributary of the Conway River, 1.8 miles from the mission. A rock-hop takes you to the far side of the stream and a nice resting spot.

 Old-Growth

 Wildflowers

Another option is to backtrack from Pocosin Mission and meet the AT. For a decent view, head left, southbound, on the AT. You travel through rocky woods on a single-track path, passing a spur to the PATC cabin. Climb rocky steps, winding through boulders on an artistically constructed trail leading to an outcrop with an easterly view a quarter mile distant from the Pocosin Fire Road. Even if you don't add these side hikes to the Pocosin Mission trek, you will be well rewarded.

🚶 MILESTONES

▶1	0.0	Pocosin Fire Road parking area at milepost 59.5
▶2	0.1	Cross Appalachian Trail
▶3	0.2	PATC Pocosin Cabin
▶4	1.0	Trail intersection and Pocosin Mission

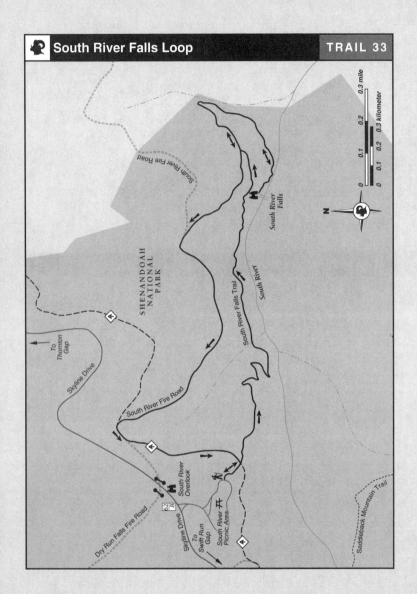

South River Falls Loop

Gravity plays a big role in this hike. Make an easy descent, and see South River Falls drop 80 feet over a rock face from a perched vista. Go farther and enjoy the view from the base of the falls. You'll have to fight the earth's tug on your climb out of the South River watershed and back to the former mountaintop pastureland, but the falls are worth the climb. This is a rich wildflower area in spring.

Best Time

Winter and spring see South River Falls at their boldest. In addition, spring wildflowers are rich in this valley. Summer offers cool deep woods. Autumn colors are worthy, but the falls flow less vigorously.

Finding the Trail

The trailhead is at South River Picnic Area at milepost 62.8 on Skyline Drive. The path starts at the back of the picnic area on the one-way loop road. The trailhead is on your right. The picnic area entrance is 2.7 miles north of the Swift Run Gap Entrance Station on Skyline Drive.

Trail Description

Leave the rear of the pleasant South River Picnic Area on a wide dirt footpath, ▶1 the South River Falls Trail, and intersect the Appalachian Trail (AT). Watch for piled rocks in this long ago overgrown farmland. Continue down to a switchback at 0.4 mile. ▶2 Twist and turn three more times before

TRAIL USE
Dayhiking

LENGTH
4.5 miles, 2–3 hours

**CUMULATIVE
ELEVATION +/-**
-1,000'/+1,000'

DIFFICULTY
– 1 2 **3** 4 5 +

TRAIL TYPE
Loop

START & FINISH
N38° 22.860'
W78° 31.021'

FEATURES
Stream
Waterfall
Wildflowers
Autumn Colors
Geologic Interest

FACILITIES
Picnic tables
Water
Restroom

Stream

Wildflowers

Geologic Interest

Waterfall

This trip is one
of the park's
better wildflower
destinations.

Wildflowers

coming to the South River, which is a small but wide creek at this point. Cross a side branch and enjoy the lush streamside environment.

Violets, toothwort, white trillium, and wild geranium color the moist margins, as do straight-trunked tulip trees and gray beeches. Other wildflowers include trout lily, false Solomon's seal, jack-in-the-pulpit, and columbine. Come to a second tributary at 0.7 mile. The valley narrows, and so does the stream. Cross a rock field at 1.0 mile, then step across a bouldery tributary. Ahead and to your right is the top of the falls, but keep going—there's a better and safer viewpoint a short distance past the granite overhang to your left. Walk out on the outcrop, bordered with a manmade stone wall to your right and see South River Falls. ▶3 It spills over a rock face and then splits into two chutes charging downward. There is so much more light here than in the dark streamside environment. South River Falls is spotlighted as well.

South River is slowly, unceasingly cutting into the precipitous stone barricade. Saddleback Mountain rises to your left. For a different perspective continue down the trail, reaching a junction at 1.4 miles. Veer right toward the base of the falls. ▶4 Curve past a tributary into a fertile wildflower zone. Notice the boundary with the Rapidan Wildlife

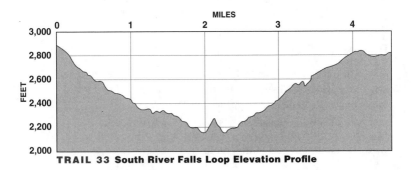

TRAIL 33 South River Falls Loop Elevation Profile

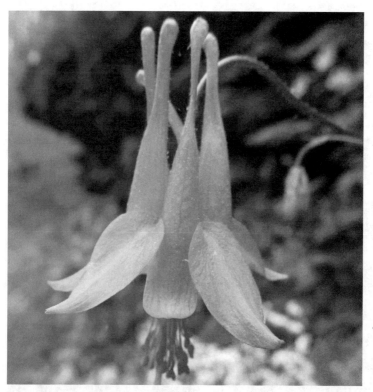

Columbine *dangles from a rock outcrop on the way to South River Falls.*

Management Area, a State of Virginia property
bordering the park. Descend to river level again
and reach a flat. Head upriver on a narrow foot
trail, passing an impressive fractured rock rampart
to your right. Stone steps aid your ascent. Come
to the base of South River Falls at 2.1 miles. ▶5
Looking up, you can clearly see the narrow chute
splitting in two before resuming a calmer path
toward the sea. This view is superior to the higher
falls perspective.

Waterfall

Yellow Birches

Yellow birch trees shade mossy rocks and ferns. Look for peeling yellowish-gold bark with horizontal stripes. Larger yellow birches peel on their upper branches not on their lower trunks. The twigs and leaves, when crushed, have a slight wintergreen aroma. Primarily a tree of the north ranging from Minnesota to Maine, yellow birches stretch down the spine of the Appalachians all the way to the South Carolina and Georgia mountain regions. They can be found in moist, cool environments throughout the mountains of Virginia.

Yellow birches often sprout on nutrient-rich rotting logs. Later, the yellow birch grows and the log rots completely away, leaving the yellow birch to look as if it grew legs.

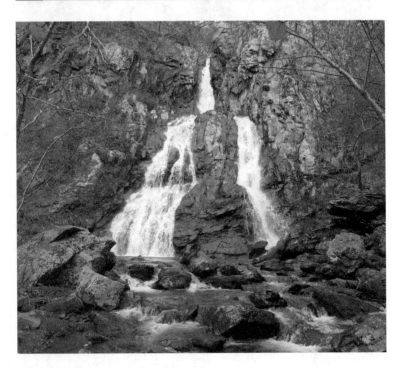

South River Falls *splits into channels as it drops.*

Finish your uphill backtracking at 2.8 miles, then veer right onto new trail, rising toward the South River Fire Road. ▶6 You can still hear the roar of South River Falls. Meet the South River Fire Road at 3.2 miles. ▶7 Turn left and continue a moderate ascent on a wide track. A lucky hiker might see yellow lady slippers hereabouts in season. Meet the AT at 4.1 miles. ▶8 Turn left here, southbound, traveling through younger woods mixed with pine on a single-track path. Complete the loop portion of the hike at 4.4 miles. Turn left on the South River Falls Trail to reach the South River Picnic Area. ▶9 Enjoy a well-deserved lunch or cookout after your hiking adventure.

 Autumn Colors

🚶 MILESTONES

▶1	0.0	South River Picnic Area
▶2	0.4	First switchback
▶3	1.3	Upper observation point of South River Falls
▶4	1.4	Right turn to base of falls
▶5	2.1	Base of South River Falls
▶6	2.8	Veer right toward South River Fire Road
▶7	3.2	Left on South River Fire Road
▶8	4.1	Left, southbound, on the AT
▶9	4.5	Return to parking area

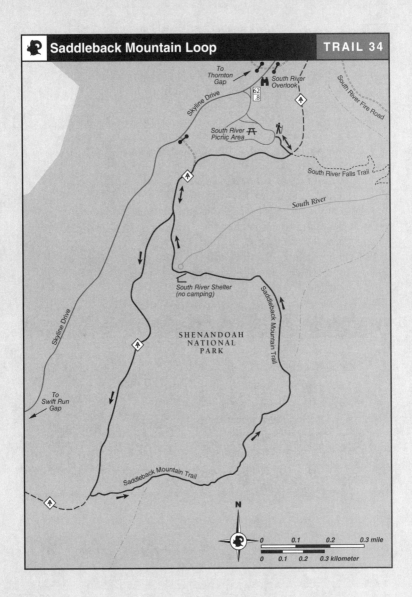

Saddleback Mountain Loop

TRAIL 34

To
Thornton
Gap

South River
Overlook

Skyline Drive

62
.8

South River
Picnic Area

South River Falls Trail

South River

South River Shelter
(no camping)

SHENANDOAH
NATIONAL
PARK

Saddleback Mountain Trail

South River Fire Road

Skyline Drive

To
Swift Run
Gap

Saddleback Mountain Trail

N

0   0.1   0.2   0.3 mile

0   0.1   0.2   0.3 kilometer

Saddleback Mountain Loop

The Appalachian Trail (AT) meanders over the crest of the Blue Ridge and provides a rewarding hiking experience through Shenandoah National Park. This long-distance path stretches well beyond the borders of the park, extending from Georgia to Maine. This particular loop allows you to enjoy a relatively level, easy stretch of the world's most famous footpath and then circle back on a seldom-used side trail that avails solitude. The elevation changes along this hike are not great, making it accessible for less able hikers or those with young families. Finally, the South River Picnic Area with picnic facilities scattered under the shade of hardwood trees, where this hike starts, makes a fine jumping-off point.

Best Time

Each season is a fine time to enjoy the subtle beauties on this lesser-hiked circuit.

Finding the Trail

The trailhead is at South River Picnic Area at milepost 62.8 on Skyline Drive. The path starts at the back of the picnic area on the one-way loop road. The South River Falls trailhead is on your right. The picnic area entrance is 2.7 miles north of Swift Run Gap Entrance Station on Skyline Drive.

Trail Description

Your hike starts on the South River Falls Trail, ▶1 a wide dirt footpath used by many to reach South River

TRAIL USE
Dayhiking,
Child-Friendly

LENGTH
3.9 miles, 2½–3½ hours

**CUMULATIVE
ELEVATION +/-**
+340'/-340'

DIFFICULTY
− 1 **2** 3 4 5 +

TRAIL TYPE
Loop

START & FINISH
N38° 22.860'
W78° 31.021'

FEATURES
Ridgeline
Autumn Colors
Wildflowers
Secluded

FACILITIES
Picnic tables
Restrooms
Water

Falls, which can be a great addition to this moderate dayhike. It's only 0.1 mile to the fabled AT. Here, this hike turns right, south, on the AT. ▶2 The surprisingly level track allows your mind to wander, contemplating your own chance at the 2,100-mile journey that a few thousand hearty souls attempt to complete each year. Most don't make it. Traditionally, AT thru-hikers have walked from south to north, reaching Shenandoah National Park sometime in late spring. However, a smaller contingency leaves Maine in June and heads south, trying to reach Georgia before the first mountain snows fall. These "southbounders" pass through Shenandoah in September.

Sporadic large oaks are mixed in with a younger forest. The pioneer trees—locusts, cherry, and pines—are relenting to maples and other hardwoods. At 0.4 mile, the AT joins an old roadbed, bearing left onto a grassy track. The walking remains easy. At 0.6 mile, reach a trail intersection and the loop portion of your hike. ▶3 The Saddleback Mountain Trail leaves left, but you stay right, still on the again-narrow AT. The trail climbs in a couple of short bursts and then reaches a high point at 1.2 miles. The actual summit of Saddleback Mountain is to your left. Saddleback Mountain gets its name from a pair of humps with a gap in the middle, a fine seat for an imaginary equestrian, a little east of where you are hiking. The locale is known for its trillium displays in early May.

 Ridgeline

Autumn Colors

Wildflowers

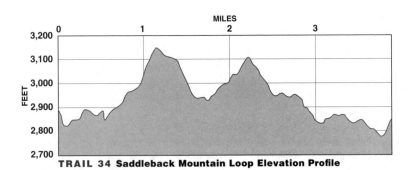

TRAIL 34 Saddleback Mountain Loop Elevation Profile

Descend past cleared trailside rocks under regal oaks and sturdy hickories. At 1.6 miles, reach the south end of the Saddleback Mountain Trail. ►4 You may have seen one or two hikers, but after you turn left and leave the AT solitude is yours. Note how the trailbed of Saddleback Mountain Trail is so faint compared to the AT. In fall wildflowers will crowd the already narrow footpath. Step over a rocky, intermittent drainage flowing off Saddleback Mountain. At 2.3 miles, the path cuts through a gap in a flat area. This is the western edge of the "saddle." Curve down the north end of the mountain, passing another flat at 2.8 miles. The downgrade continues.

 Secluded

 Wildflowers

At 3.1 miles, reach the old South River Shelter. ►5 The stone and wood building is now closed for camping and is used as a maintenance building by the Potomac Appalachian Trail Club, which maintains the AT through Shenandoah and beyond. Picnic tables make it an alluring stopping point. Continue past the rocked-in spring serving the shelter (a few steps downhill from the trail). This upwelling is the headwaters of the South River.

Amble on down a wide track to again meet the AT at 3.3 miles. ►6 You have completed the loop portion of the hike. From here, backtrack on the AT, northbound, reaching the South River Falls Trail at 3.8 miles. ►7 Turn left and reach the South River Picnic Area and the trailhead. ►8

🚶	**MILESTONES**	
►1	0.0	South River Picnic Area
►2	0.1	Right on the AT
►3	0.6	Saddleback Mountain Trail leaves left; stay with the AT
►4	1.6	Left on Saddleback Mountain Trail
►5	3.1	PATC maintenance shelter
►6	3.3	Right on the AT
►7	3.8	Left on South River Falls Trail
►8	3.9	South River Picnic Area

CHAPTER 3

South District

35. Hightop

36. Rocky Mount Loop

37. Rocky Mountain Loop

38. Loft Mountain Loop

39. Patterson Ridge Loop

40. Big Run Loop

41. Rockytop and Big Run Loop

42. Austin Mountain and Madison Run Loop

43. Falls Loop from Browns Gap

44. Furnace Mountain via Blackrock

45. Blackrock Loop

46. Big Branch Falls via Moormans River

47. Chimney Rock

48. Chimney Rock via Riprap Hollow

49. Turk Mountain

50. Turk Branch Loop

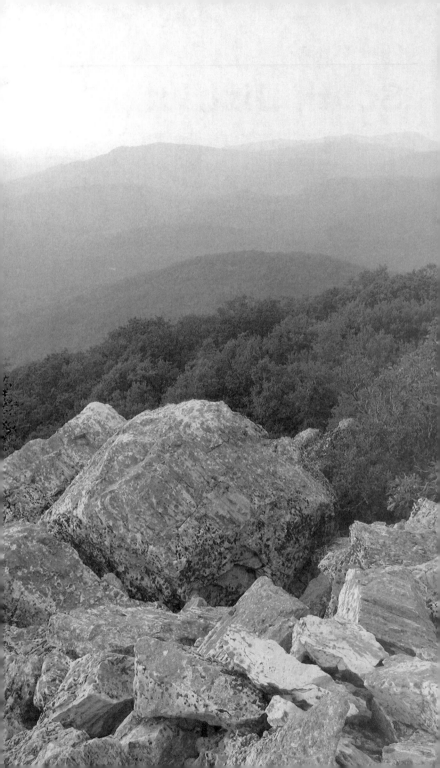

South District

The South District is the least visited of the park's three districts. Partly because it is more distant from the Washington metroplex, the South District has a more relaxed, remote aura. It also has the fewest visitor facilities, which are limited to the Loft Mountain area, with a camp store and campground, and Dundo Picnic Area, a few miles south of Loft Mountain. US 33 connecting Elkton to Stanardsville marks the north end of the South District. The district stretches south to Rockfish Gap near Waynesboro, connected by 40 miles of Skyline Drive.

The South District has many characteristics that separate it from the others. First, it has the largest acreage of designated wilderness. It also is the lowest in elevation but is the rockiest parcel of this boulder-laden park. It has the park's biggest stream—Big Run. The trails here are the least hiked, especially if you get off the Appalachian Trail (AT).

Hiking opportunities are numerous and varied in length, difficulty, and destination. Heading south from Swift Run Gap, you can first hike to Hightop, where a wildflower-bordered track rises to outcrops with westerly vistas limited only by the clarity of the sky. Both Rocky Mount and Rocky Mountain are quartz-tipped mountain crests divided by steep drainages where translucent streams gurgle through wild corridors. They offer secluded trekking experiences.

Enjoy more views from Loft Mountain, as well as human history and the convenience of incorporating park facilities into a hike. Saunter among the pines on Patterson Ridge on a challenging loop that travels high and low. Big Run Loop takes you from Skyline Drive to the upper Big Run watershed before using the AT to close the loop.

Rockytop Mountain not only recalls the University of Tennessee fight song of the same name but also lives up to it name. Incredible and nearly continuous views characterize this fire-scarred, stone-pocked ridge. Lower Big Run is a wild stream with big pools, rapids, and plenty of room to roam. Austin Mountain is another rocky crest that is pimpled with evergreens and

Overleaf and opposite: A boulder field *provides an excellent view from atop Turk Mountain (Trail 49).*

laden with views of the surrounding terrain in a solitude unimagined elsewhere in the park. The Falls Loop from Browns Gap drops off the east side of the Blue Ridge and makes a circuit along two waterfall-rich streams in Doyles River and Jones Run. Old-growth trees on Jones Run are an added treat.

Furnace Mountain is one of those hidden gems passed over by most hikers. Conversely, Blackrock, a geological wonder, is a popular peak that presents spectacular landscapes from its boulder garden summit. Farther south, Moormans River marks distant terrain, with Big Branch Falls a highlight. Hikers can access Chimney Rock, with its first-rate views from either Riprap Hollow, where falls and pools ease a climb, or from Skyline Drive, where you travel rocky terrain from the AT, running the spine of South District.

Turk Mountain is one peak almost everyone can bag. And the vistas from there are simply stunning. Turk Branch offers a chance to explore the back of beyond in solitude and on your own terms. Put together the hikes here, whether loops or out-and-backs, present the best of the South District.

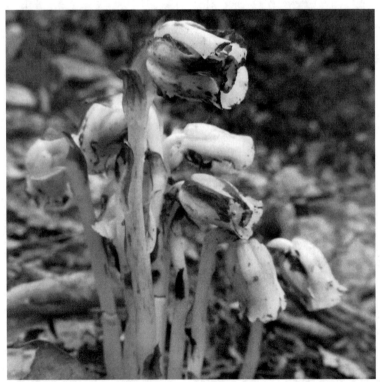

Indian ghost pipe *emerges from the late summer forest floor.*

Permits

Permits are not required for dayhiking. Backpackers must get a backcountry permit to stay in the backcountry. Simple self-registration stations are located at Swift Run Gap Entrance Station, Loft Mountain Wayside, and Rockfish Gap Entrance Station.

Maps

For the South District, here are the USGS 7.5-minute (1:24,000-scale) topographic quadrangles that you will need, listed in the order that you will need them as you hike along your route.

Trail 35: *Swift Run Gap*
Trail 36: *McGaheysville*
Trail 37: *McGaheysville*
Trail 38: *McGaheysville*
Trail 39: *McGaheysville*
Trail 40: *McGaheysville* and *Browns Cove*
Trail 41: *Browns Cove* and *McGaheysville*
Trail 42: *Browns Cove, McGaheysville,* and *Grottoes*
Trail 43: *Browns Cove*
Trail 44: *Browns Cove* and *Crimora*
Trail 45: *Browns Cove*
Trail 46: *Browns Cove*
Trail 47: *Crimora*
Trail 48: *Crimora*
Trail 49: *Crimora* and *Waynesboro East*
Trail 50: *Crimora* and *Waynesboro East*

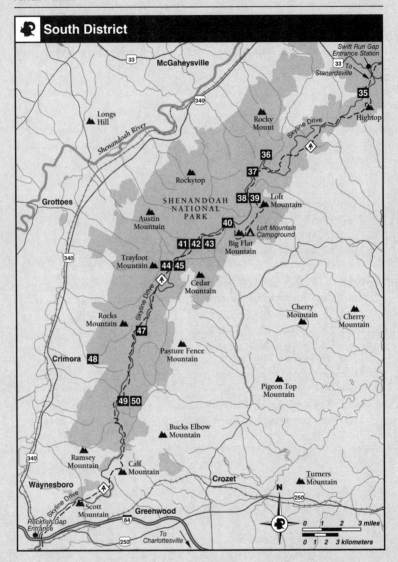

South District

TRAIL FEATURES TABLE

South District

TRAIL	Difficulty	Length	Type	USES & ACCESS	TERRAIN	NATURE	OTHER
35	3	3.2	Out & Back	Dayhiking, Backpacking	Summit	Autumn Colors, Wildflowers	Great Views, Geologic Interest
36	5	9.8	Loop	Dayhiking, Backpacking	Summit, Ridgeline, Stream	Autumn Colors, Wildflowers	Great Views, Geologic Interest, Historic Interest
37	5	9.5	Loop	Dayhiking, Backpacking	Ridgeline, Stream, Waterfall	Autumn Colors	Great Views, Geologic Interest, Swimming, Steep
38	2	2.9	Loop	Dayhiking, Pets Prohibited	Ridgeline	Autumn Colors, Wildflowers	Great Views, Geologic Interest
39	5	9.7	Loop	Dayhiking, Backpacking	Ridgeline, Stream	Autumn Colors, Wildflowers	Great Views, Swimming, Secluded
40	3	5.8	Loop	Dayhiking	Ridgeline, Stream	Autumn Colors, Wildflowers	Great Views, Geologic Interest, Historic Interest
41	5	13.3	Loop	Dayhiking, Backpacking	Ridgeline, Stream	Autumn Colors	Great Views, Historic Interest, Swimming, Secluded, Steep
42	4	8.8	Loop	Dayhiking, Backpacking	Ridgeline, Stream	Autumn Colors, Wildflowers	Great Views, Historic Interest
43	4	7.0	Loop	Dayhiking, Backpacking	Ridgeline, Stream, Waterfall	Autumn Colors, Wildflowers, Old-Growth	Geologic Interest, Historic Interest
44	3	6.8	Out & Back	Dayhiking, Backpacking	Summit, Ridgeline	Autumn Colors	Great Views, Geologic Interest, Secluded
45	1	1.1	Loop	Dayhiking, Child-Friendly	Summit, Ridgeline	Autumn Colors	Great Views, Geologic Interest
46	4	7.6	Out & Back	Dayhiking, Backpacking	Stream, Waterfall	Autumn Colors, Wildflowers	Swimming, Secluded
47	2	3.2	Out & Back	Dayhiking, Backpacking	Ridgeline	Autumn Colors	Great Views, Geologic Interest
48	4	6.8	Out & Back	Dayhiking	Ridgeline, Stream, Waterfall	Autumn Colors, Wildflowers	Great Views, Swimming
49	2	2.4	Out & Back	Dayhiking	Summit, Ridgeline	Autumn Colors	Great Views, Geologic Interest, Secluded
50	4	7.5	Loop	Dayhiking, Backpacking	Ridgeline, Stream, Waterfall	Autumn Colors, Wildflowers	Historic Interest, Secluded

USES & ACCESS
- Dayhiking
- Backpacking
- Child-Friendly
- Pets Prohibited

TYPE
- Loop
- Out & Back

DIFFICULTY
- 1 2 3 4 5 +
- less   more

TERRAIN
- Summit
- Ridgeline
- Stream
- Waterfall

NATURE
- Autumn Colors
- Wildflowers
- Wildlife
- Old-Growth

FEATURES
- Great Views
- Geologic Interest
- Historic Interest
- Swimming
- Secluded
- Steep

South District

TRAIL 35

Dayhiking, Backpacking
3.2 miles, Out & Back
Difficulty: 1 **2** 3 4 5

Hightop 243
Get a taste of the Appalachian Trail while climbing
one of the South District's higher mountains. Just at
the point where novice hikers get tired of climbing,
the path tops out and presents a very rewarding
view. In late spring, the trailside woods are carpeted
with trillium and other wildflowers.

TRAIL 36

Dayhiking, Backpacking
9.8 miles, Loop
Difficulty: 1 2 3 4 **5**

Rocky Mount Loop 247
If you like wilderness hiking in solitude, take this
ambitious loop. Leave the Blue Ridge to access the
summit of Rocky Mount for far-reaching panoramas. Descend sharply to Gap Run. Return up the
watershed to the Rocky Mount Trail, completing the
circuit. You'll have this untamed slice of Shenandoah
to yourself.

TRAIL 37

Dayhiking, Backpacking
9.5 miles, Loop
Difficulty: 1 2 3 4 **5**

Rocky Mountain Loop 253
This loop explores varied natural environments
enhanced with copious vistas. Traverse Rocky
Mountain amid scenery reminiscent of the West
before reaching the park's largest watercourse, Big
Run. Follow Big Run and Rocky Mountain Run back
to the high country.

Loft Mountain Loop 259

TRAIL 38

Dayhiking,
Pets Prohibited
2.9 miles, Loop
Difficulty: 1 **2** 3 4 5

This gentle trek takes the Frazier Discovery Trail to a massive rock outcrop with an extensive view. Here Loft Mountain opens to the heavens above and the lowlands below. Beyond the vista, pick up the Appalachian Trail, southward through a transitional forest to meet a paved path near the Loft Mountain Campground camp store. Easily descend back to the trailhead.

Patterson Ridge Loop 265

TRAIL 39

Dayhiking, Backpacking
9.7 miles, Loop
Difficulty: 1 2 3 4 **5**

This tough loop unites a remote wilderness trail, the park's biggest stream, some high country, and a campground. The infrequently hiked Patterson Ridge Trail descends to Big Run. Rock-hop your way along the watercourse, then climb to Skyline Drive. Join the fabled Appalachian Trail, heading northbound passing near Loft Mountain Campground.

Big Run Loop 271

TRAIL 40

Dayhiking
5.8 miles, Loop
Difficulty: 1 2 **3** 4 5

Explore several types of forest and mountain lands. Leave Big Run Overlook, and head into prototype oak woods. Travel a dry piney ridgeline with its attendant mountain laurel. Make your way to a moist valley harboring cove hardwoods. Join the Appalachian Trail and the spine of the Blue Ridge, hiking amid boulder fields and bluffs.

Rockytop and Big Run Loop 277

TRAIL 41

Dayhiking, Backpacking
13.3 miles, Loop
Difficulty: 1 2 3 4 **5**

Ramble the high ridge of Rockytop Mountain where talus slopes and open boulders make for solitude-filled lookouts of the adjacent mountainscape and Shenandoah Valley beyond. Drop into crystalline Big Run, exploring the gorgeous valley of the park's largest watershed from low to high.

TRAIL 42

Dayhiking, Backpacking
8.8 miles, Loop
Difficulty: 1 2 3 **4** 5

Austin Mountain and
Madison Run Loop 283

Leave historic Browns Gap, tracing a modernized toll path, joining Austin Mountain Trail. Hike past clearings and over several talus slopes, availing seldom-seen outstanding views. Descend in pines to Madison Run, where rich forest shades a trout stream. Trek up the valley, winding along ridges and hollows back to Browns Gap.

TRAIL 43

Dayhiking, Backpacking
7.0 miles, Loop
Difficulty: 1 2 3 **4** 5

Falls Loop from Browns Gap 289

Water lovers will fall for this loop. The trail passes three major cataracts and numerous other cascades as it explores two boulder-strewn canyons connected by the Appalachian Trail. The hike up Jones Run passes some old-growth tulip trees with impressive girths.

TRAIL 44

Dayhiking, Backpacking
6.8 miles, Out & Back
Difficulty: 1 2 **3** 4 5

Furnace Mountain via Blackrock.... 295

This geologically rich hike visits huge outcrops and open talus slopes where rocks by the thousands carpet the mountainsides. First, soak in the outstanding views of Blackrock Summit with others, then a rocky trail leads to the solitude of Furnace Mountain and a fine vista.

TRAIL 45

Dayhiking,
Child-Friendly
1.1 miles, Loop
Difficulty: **1** 2 3 4 5

Blackrock Loop 301

Start at nearly 3,000 feet, and hike to an incredible rock jumble on the Appalachian Trail. Views extend for miles in multiple directions from the summit of Blackrock. After gaining views from several spots, reenter woods, and work your way back to the trailhead.

Big Branch Falls via Moormans River 305

TRAIL 46

Dayhiking, Backpacking
7.6 miles, Out & Back
Difficulty: 1 2 3 **4** 5

This is perhaps the most bypassed, ignored, and undervisited trail-accessible waterfall in all of Shenandoah National Park. First, descend to the North Fork Moormans River, with cascades and pools in a deep valley bordered by high ridges. Finally, climb along low-flow Big Branch, with its open watery bowls divided by rock slabs where the stream falls in slide cascades.

Chimney Rock 309

TRAIL 47

Dayhiking, Backpacking
3.2 miles, Out & Back
Difficulty: 1 **2** 3 4 5

Take the Appalachian Trail under oaks to rocky Riprap Trail. Cruise past a stony vista, and then hike past boulder gardens to reach Chimney Rock, a distended stone spire presenting views of the adjacent talus-covered peaks and Shenandoah Valley beyond.

Chimney Rock via Riprap Hollow . . . 315

TRAIL 48

Dayhiking
6.8 miles, Out & Back
Difficulty: 1 2 3 **4** 5

Bring your camera with you on this hike. Tramp up Riprap Hollow, where the environment goes through dramatic changes. Start in a lush streamside forest, then slice through a narrow canyon to a deep swimming hole. Open onto a piney, rocky hillside. Emerge onto Rocks Mountain with its views from airy, quartz outcrops, culminating in Chimney Rock.

TRAIL 49

Dayhiking
2.4 miles, Out & Back
Difficulty: 1 **2** 3 4 5

Turk Mountain 321

Hike to a boulder-strewn summit. This dead-end trek rises from quiet Turk Gap. Wander woodland to emerge at the crest of Turk Mountain, where a huge talus slope opens the sky to limitless western vistas of Shenandoah Valley.

TRAIL 50

Dayhiking, Backpacking
7.5 miles, Loop
Difficulty: 1 2 3 **4** 5

Turk Branch Loop 325

Wander the park's most southerly and seemingly most forgotten reaches. Descend along remote Turk Branch, passing old homesites. Head up South Fork Moormans River Valley to meet the Appalachian Trail. Turn north on Shenandoah's master path, gaining limited views amid the pines and oaks before returning to Turk Gap.

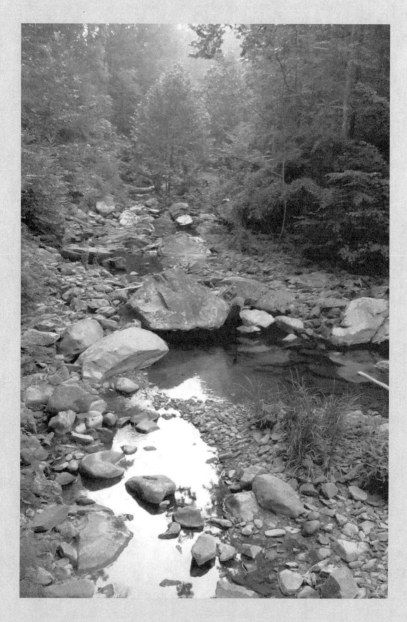

Morning light *breaks on North Fork Moormans River en route to Big Branch Falls (Trail 46).*

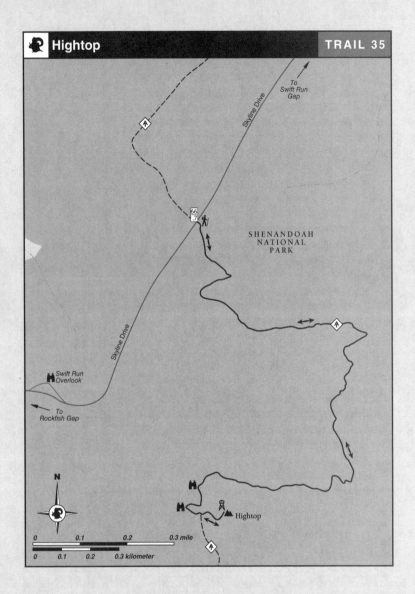

Hightop

TRAIL 35

To Swift Run Gap

Skyline Drive

SHENANDOAH NATIONAL PARK

Skyline Drive

Swift Run Overlook

To Rockfish Gap

N

Hightop

0   0.1   0.2   0.3 mile
0   0.1   0.2   0.3 kilometer

Hightop

This is one peak almost everyone can bag. Just at the point where novice hikers get tired of climbing, the path tops out and presents a very rewarding view. Get a taste of the Appalachian Trail (AT) while climbing one of the park's higher mountains.

Best Time

Fall through spring is optimal for this hike. You can enjoy wildflowers and far-reaching views in spring. Summer can be hazy. Fall has colors and clarity of sky. Winter offers clear days and sure solitude.

Finding the Trail

The Hightop Mountain parking area is located at milepost 66.7 on Skyline Drive. From the Swift Run Gap Entrance Station, drive south on Skyline Drive for 1.2 miles to the parking area on your right.

Trail Description

Start the trek by crossing Skyline Drive from the Hightop Mountain parking area. ▶1 Pick up the AT, southbound. Hike through a bramble- and briar-covered area on a moderate uphill grade. This area is transitioning from field to forest. Enter woods and pass two large gray boulders acting as sentinels for the mountaintop ahead. Ahead, more lichen-covered boulders line the path, which becomes rocky as it climbs. The adjacent woods can be rocky too. Step over a gurgling spring branch that runs dry by fall. Cross an older and steeper trail

TRAIL USE
Dayhiking, Backpacking

LENGTH
3.2 miles, 2–3 hours

**CUMULATIVE
ELEVATION +/-**
+950'/-950'

DIFFICULTY
– 1 2 **3** 4 5 +

TRAIL TYPE
Out & Back

START & FINISH
N38° 20.713'
W78° 33.178'

FEATURES
Summit
Autumn Colors
Wildflowers
Geologic Interest
Great Views

FACILITIES
None

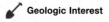 **Geologic Interest**

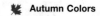 **Autumn Colors**

at 0.5 mile—good thing that way to the top was abandoned. ▶2

This side of Hightop is a rich wildflower area in spring. Expect to see white trillium, as well as the overhanging maroon blooms of Catesby's trillium. Other wildflowers you may see include wild geranium, may apples, and star chickweed. A level section ahead offers a brief reprieve before the AT starts switchbacking up the mountain at a steeper grade. At mile 1.0, the trail again levels. ▶3 The larger oak and tulip trees at this elevation take on a gnarled appearance; the weather can be rough up here and the trees show it. But nature has a gentler side on Hightop too that is evident by its verdant fertility in early spring (May and early June).

The AT swings around the right side of Hightop, soon passing two outcrops that offer first-rate vistas. The first outcrop, at 1.4 miles, reveals Massanutten Peak straight ahead. ▶4 To your right is the town of Elkton, and of course, the Shenandoah Valley stretches out below. North Mountain is in the farthest distance and can be seen on clear days. The cluster of houses just below is the community of Sandy Bottom.

The next outcrop, also to the right of the trail, is clearly more spectacular and a just reward for your efforts. ▶5 The rock face of Rocky Mount stands

 Wildflowers

This is one peak that almost everyone can bag.

Great Views

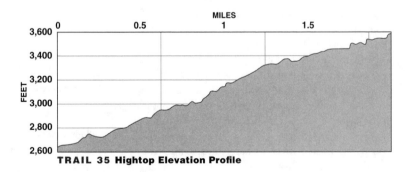

TRAIL 35 Hightop Elevation Profile

plainly visible. The bulk of Shenandoah's mountains extend in wave upon wave in the distance. The mass to your left is Flattop Mountain. Skyline Drive flows just below you.

Great Views

Continue a short distance farther until you come to a trace of a trail leading left. A concrete signpost indicates the AT leaving right and downhill for Hightop trail hut, then on down to Georgia. Consider visiting the hut if you want to add 1.2 miles to your hike. Follow the trail left and quickly get to the level top of Hightop, at 3,587 feet, at mile 1.6. ►6 Views are limited here since the fire tower was dismantled, but it makes a good lunch spot if the winds are high or the sun excessively strong on the outcrops. From the trailhead you gained nearly 1,000 feet of altitude in less than 2 miles.

Summit

🚶	**MILESTONES**	
►1	0.0	Hightop parking area at milepost 66.7
►2	0.5	Old steep track crosses the AT
►3	1.0	Gap
►4	1.4	First outcrop with views
►5	1.5	Second outcrop with spectacular views
►6	1.6	Hightop Peak

Rocky Mount Loop

TRAIL 36

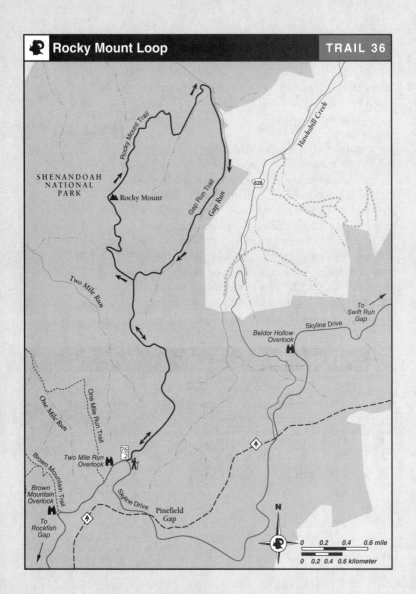

SHENANDOAH
NATIONAL
PARK

Rocky Mount Trail

▲ Rocky Mount

Gap Run Trail

Gap Run

Hawksbill Creek

628

Two Mile Run

To
Swift Run
Gap

Beldor Hollow
Overlook

Skyline Drive

One Mile Run

One Mile Run Trail

76
2

Two Mile Run
Overlook

Brown Mountain Trail

Brown
Mountain
Overlook

To
Rockfish
Gap

Skyline Drive

Pinefield
Gap

N

| 0 | 0.2 | 0.4 | 0.6 mile |

| 0 | 0.2 | 0.4 | 0.6 kilometer |

Rocky Mount Loop

If you like wilderness hiking in solitude, take this ambitious loop. Leave the main crest of the Blue Ridge to access the summit of Rocky Mount for far-reaching views. Descend sharply to Gap Run and return up the watershed to the Rocky Mount Trail. You'll have this untamed slice of Shenandoah to yourself.

Best Time

You will experience solitude just about any time of year. Spring offers extensive views as well as wildflowers along Gap Run. Summer can be hazy and sometimes warm. Fall sports colors and clear skies again. Winter is a good time too, especially after fronts, when the air is crisp and translucent.

Finding the Trail

The trailhead can be found 0.1 mile north of Two Mile Run Overlook, at milepost 76.2 on Skyline Drive. It is 10.7 miles south of the Swift Run Gap Entrance Station, on the west side of Skyline Drive.

Trail Description

Be careful walking along Skyline Drive to the trail's beginning. ►1 Rocky Mount Trail starts at the north end of the rock wall stretching from Two Mile Run Overlook. Immediately climb a wooded knoll before dropping northeast on a narrow ridge. The lightly used single-track foot trail alternately dips and levels off in oak-dominated woods before coming

TRAIL USE
Dayhiking, Backpacking

LENGTH
9.8 miles, 6–7 hours

CUMULATIVE ELEVATION +/-
+2,200'/-2,200'

DIFFICULTY
– 1 2 3 4 **5** +

TRAIL TYPE
Loop

START & FINISH
N38° 17.942'
W78° 38.821'

FEATURES
Ridgeline
Summit
Stream
Autumn Colors
Wildflowers
Geologic Interest
Great Views
Historic Interest

FACILITIES
None

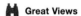 **Ridgeline**

to a saddle at 0.7 mile. Veer to the left, southwest, side of the ridge among pine woods. To your left are intermittent views of Rocky Mountain (not to be confused with Rocky Mount) between scads of mountain laurel. You can also possibly look back at your car at Two Mile Run Overlook.

At 1.1 miles, come to a gap, ▶2 then swing around the northeast end of an unnamed knob. The valley of Hawksbill Creek drops far below. The forest changes to birch trees with a high canopy. Descend to rejoin the ridgecrest at 1.6 miles. Continue downhill. Rocky Mount lurks ever higher through the trees ahead. Reach another gap and a trail junction at 2.2 miles. ▶3 To your right is Gap Run Trail, your return route.

Continue straight on Rocky Mount Trail, beginning your 800-foot climb up the south face of Rocky Mount. Look between the oaks, pines, and azaleas lining the path back at Two Mile Run Overlook. The hollow of Two Mile Run lies below. Cross a partly forested talus slope at 2.6 miles and then switchback. Twice you think you're nearing the summit, but the stony trail keeps snaking through rocks and boulders.

Geologic Interest

Come to a side trail on your left just before reaching the true top of Rocky Mount at 3.3 miles. ▶4 It leads to a pine-framed outcrop with stunning views. A white quartz wall runs to your left. Look out over

Great Views

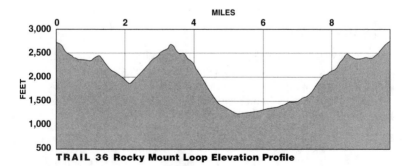

TRAIL 36 Rocky Mount Loop Elevation Profile

Two Mile Run. At the head of the run stands Two Mile Run Overlook, where you started, and the crest of the Blue Ridge. One Mile Run cuts the next valley south. Rocky Mountain rises beyond that. To your right stretches the South Fork Shenandoah River and the farms and fields that surround it.

Climb a bit, then reach the wooded peak of Rocky Mount (2,741 feet). The now lesser-used trail drops along the base of a huge granite slope. Continue descending through a heavily canopied forest before coming to a pine stand with views into Gap Run. On a switchback, the rocky slope of Beldor Ridge is visible directly ahead. Traverse a rock field at mile 4.4, and reach a tributary of Gap Run at 4.6 miles. ▶5 Rock-hop the streamlet, dotted with pale rocks, twice in succession. Make a sharp right turn into a clearing before reaching Gap Run at 5.3 miles. ▶6 This is an easy rock-hop during normal flows. A concrete signpost stands on the far side of the creek. It is 0.7 mile downstream to the park boundary.

Turn right on Gap Run Trail, gently ascending an old road that has been washed out in places. Look for black birch shading this cooler, moister vale. Backpackers find legal campsites in the flats of Gap Run. Pass a clearing, once a homesite, worth exploring, and come to a second signpost at mile 5.5. There is a real aura of isolation here, even though this valley was once peopled.

Stay on the roadbed, and enter the rock-strewn flood plain of Gap Run. Overflow channels braid the woods, leaving the exact path unclear. Look for blue paint blazes marking the trail, and pick up the road-bed again, coming to another trail signpost at mile 6.0. ▶7 An old road leaves the park left. Dogwoods and white pines are sprinkled throughout the young forest, which was a field when this park was established. Turn right and travel along Gap Run, crossing the creek and its tributaries easily.

Summit

Stream

Historic Interest

Wildflowers

Stream

Cross Gap Run a final time at 7.2 miles. ▶8 The trail grade sharpens, and Gap Run Trail follows a stony, dry wash toward a low spot on Rocky Mount Trail. Leave the dry wash at a switchback, and surge upward a short distance, reaching the gap at 7.6 miles. ▶9 You were here before. Turn left on Rocky Mount Trail, and retrace your steps 2.2 miles back to Skyline Drive and the Blue Ridge. ▶10

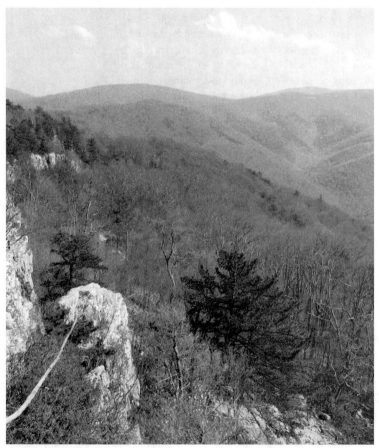

Looking back *to Two Mile Run Overlook from the top of Rocky Mount*

MILESTONES

▶1	0.0	Two Mile Run Overlook at milepost 76.2
▶2	1.1	Gap
▶3	2.2	At gap and Gap Run Trail, stay left on Rocky Mount Trail
▶4	3.3	Vista and then summit of Rocky Mount
▶5	4.6	Tributary of Gap Run
▶6	5.3	Reach and cross Gap Run
▶7	6.0	Old road leaves left at post; Gap Run Trail stays right
▶8	7.2	Cross Gap Run a final time
▶9	7.6	At end of Gap Run Trail, stay left on Rocky Mount Trail
▶10	9.8	Two Mile Run Overlook at milepost 76.2

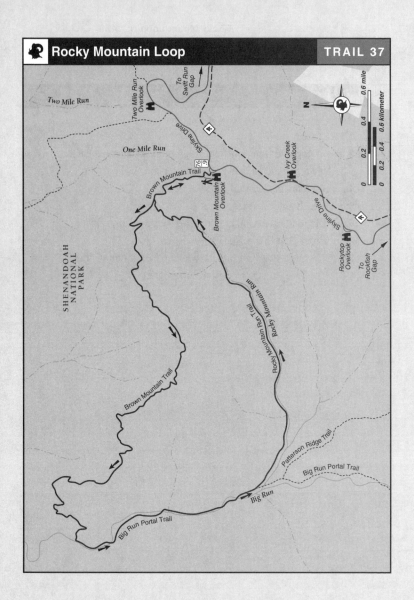

Rocky Mountain Loop

TRAIL 37

Two Mile Run

One Mile Run

Two Mile Run Overlook

To Swift Run Gap

Skyline Drive

76
9

Brown Mountain Trail

Brown Mountain Overlook

Ivy Creek Overlook

Skyline Drive

Rockytop Overlook

To Rockfish Gap

SHENANDOAH NATIONAL PARK

Brown Mountain Trail

Rocky Mountain Run Trail

Rocky Mountain Run

Patterson Ridge Trail

Big Run Portal Trail

Big Run

Big Run Portal Trail

N

0.2   0.4   0.6 mile

0.2   0.4   0.6 kilometer

0   0

Rocky Mountain Loop

This challenging hike entails a lot of ups and downs; this loop explores varied natural environments enhanced with copious vistas. Bring your camera. Take the Brown Mountain Trail, passing over Rocky Mountain and scenery reminiscent of the West, with stone spires rising from the forest before ending up at the park's largest watercourse, Big Run. Follow Big Run and Rocky Mountain Run back to the high country. *Note that the first half of this hike is dry and that fording Big Run can be hazardous in high water.*

In the South District, you have Rockytop, Rocky Mount, and Rocky Mountain all adjacent to one another. The names can be confusing, but each ridgeline presents distinct and scenic hiking opportunities. On this hike you are on Rocky Mountain, yet looking out on Rocky Mount and Rockytop.

TRAIL USE
Dayhiking, Backpacking

LENGTH
9.5 miles, 6–7½ hours

CUMULATIVE ELEVATION +/-
1,580'/-1,580'

DIFFICULTY
– 1 2 3 4 **5** +

TRAIL TYPE
Loop

START & FINISH
N38° 17.543'
W78° 39.480'

FEATURES
Ridgeline
Stream
Autumn Colors
Geologic Interest
Waterfall
Great Views
Steep
Swimming

FACILITIES
None

Best Time

This loop requires crossing unbridged Big Run and Rocky Mountain Run numerous times, and therefore it is best done when the streams are lower—late spring through late fall and before the chills of winter make stream crossings numbing. Try to time your hikes after fronts clear the skies for views from Rocky Mountain and Brown Mountain. However, summer is best for splashing in the waters of Big Run.

Finding the Trail

The hike starts at the center of Brown Mountain Overlook at milepost 76.9 on Skyline Drive.

Trail Description

Experience Shenandoah at its wildest.

Leave Brown Mountain Overlook behind, ▶1 and steeply descend through a low clearing that opens to Rocky Mountain across the gap to your west and Big Run below. Rocky Mount stands to the north, and Rockytop forms a wall to the south. Leave the low-slung sumac and locust at 0.1 mile, entering full-blown hardwoods. The track switchbacks a narrow ridgeline to reach a gap and trail junction at 0.6 mile. ▶2 To your left is the terminus of the Rocky Mountain Run Trail, your return route.

Ridgeline

Continue straight on the Brown Mountain Trail, climbing the eastern flank of Rocky Mountain amid chestnut oaks. Achieve the ridgetop via switchbacks at 1.0 mile, passing through pines. The trail begins undulating along the stony spine of Rocky Mountain, emerging at a giant quartz outcrop at 1.5 miles. ▶3 You can plainly see the crest of the Blue Ridge and Brown Mountain Overlook across the gulf of Rocky Mountain Run. Below, Big Run falls deeply beneath. Waves of mountains roll southward. This vista could be a rewarding 3-mile out-and-back endeavor if the whole loop is too ambitious.

Great Views

Autumn Colors

Beyond the outcrop, the stony track descends along the north side of Rocky Mountain under oaks, black gum, and hickory. At 2.5 miles, the now-sandy trail enters scattered pines standing over the

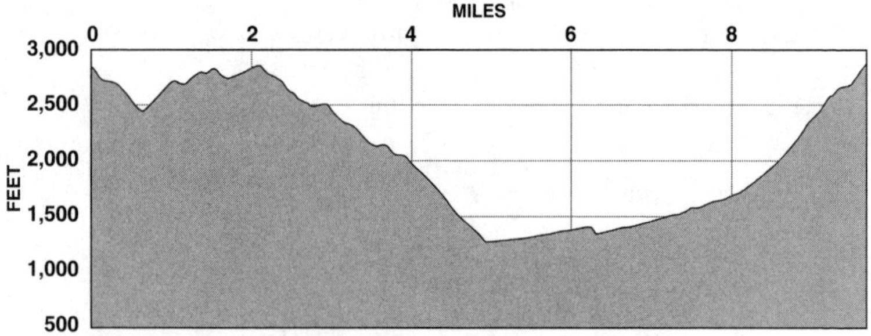

TRAIL 37 Rocky Mountain Loop Elevation Profile

low brush of blueberries. Views open. Massanutten Peak is dead ahead. Continue along the ridge, and top out on wooded Brown Mountain at mile 3.2.

Prepare for some of the finest scenery in Shenandoah National Park. Begin an irregular descent with many vistas. You'll have trouble keeping your balance on this rock-strewn trail as it switchbacks among pine and mountain laurel down the face of Brown Mountain. Why? There are multiple distracting views: Rocky Mountain, Rockytop, Big Run, Massanutten Peak, and Shenandoah Valley. Short spur trails lead to pine-framed outcrops and these views. At 3.5 miles, the trail regains the crest 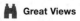 **Great Views** of the ridge. At 3.7 miles, hike downhill into a slope of patchy pines surviving between rock slabs. ▶4 Here, gaze across Bearwallow Hollow at great stone protuberances on the far ridge. At 4.1 miles, the path curves into Big Run valley. The dry west-facing slope of sporadic pines, oaks, and blueberries

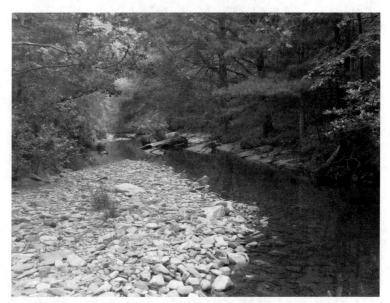

Big Run *flows crystalline along a gravel bar.*

FLORA

Shagbark Hickories

Shagbark hickories look like what their name implies, a tree with loose-plated bark sloughing off the main trunk, looking like they could use a trim, much like shaggy haired humans. The loose bark plates run vertically up the trunk of the tree.

Shagbark hickories once were an important food source for aboriginal Virginians, who sought out their surprisingly sweet nuts. Although the tree's nut production varies wildly from year to year, their thin shell and substantial nutmeat make shagbark hickory nuts an attractive choice. The best time to collect the mast was soon after the acorns fell and before the first frost of autumn. Birds and mammals competed with the Indians for the sought-after nuts, especially in years when the shagbarks produced fewer nuts.

These hickories also helped the Indians obtain food another way. Tribes fashioned the strong wood into bows to hunt game. The shagbark hickories you see here may seem like mere shade trees, but they have been a good food source for the peoples—and the beasts—of Shenandoah.

affords views of white columnar spires, and the scree slopes of Rocky Top and Big Run Portal rise from the greenery.

The white noise of Big Run resonates below as you repeatedly switchback down the stony path. Reach a concrete trail signpost, turn left, walk a few feet, and come to a second trail signpost at 4.9 miles. ▶5 Stay left at the second trail marker, joining the Big Run Portal Trail. Traverse dense forest on a foot-friendly former fire road, then rock-hop Big Run, with its small pools and noisy cascades at 5.1 miles. Alder bushes flank the trout stream, while witch hazel and sycamore shade gravel bars. Dogwoods add springtime color to the gorge. Make a second crossing at 5.6 miles. This crossing, like all the others in this watershed, can be dry-footed at normal water levels but is challenging when the water is

Stream

Swimming

high. Look for large white pines along the run. The evergreens have long, blue-green needles and evenly spaced branches. The gray vertically peeling trunks of shagbark hickories are also easy to spot.

Make two easy crossings of Big Run in succession, then reach a trail junction at 6.3 miles. ▶6 Veer left on the Rocky Mountain Run Trail. It moderately ascends an old roadbed along Rocky Mountain Run, flanked with white pine, into a more intimate valley than Big Run. The path curves easterly at 6.7 miles. Normally dry tributaries bisect the path. Make your first easy crossing of Rocky Mountain Run at 7.2 miles. Watch for a slide cascade and plunge pool on your right at 7.7 miles. ▶7

Cross Rocky Mountain Run twice at 7.8 miles, and soon leave the roadbed. Large white oaks and tulip trees stand proudly overhead. Step over a tributary of Rocky Mountain Run at 8.0 miles. Look left here as the main stream flows over a rock slab. The trail steepens and enters young spindly forest in a series of switchbacks, making a gap and trail junction at 8.9 miles. ▶8 Turn right on the Brown Mountain Trail, and retrace your steps 0.6 mile farther, back to Brown Mountain Overlook at 9.5 miles. ▶9

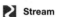 Stream

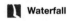 Waterfall

🚶	**MILESTONES**	
▶1	0.0	Brown Mountain Overlook at milepost 76.9
▶2	0.6	Rocky Mountain Run Trail leaves left
▶3	1.5	Great views from quartz outcrop
▶4	3.7	Vista across Bearwallow Hollow
▶5	4.9	Left on Big Run Portal Trail
▶6	6.3	Left on Rocky Mountain Run Trail
▶7	7.7	Waterfall
▶8	8.9	Right on Brown Mountain Trail
▶9	9.5	Brown Mountain Overlook at milepost 76.9

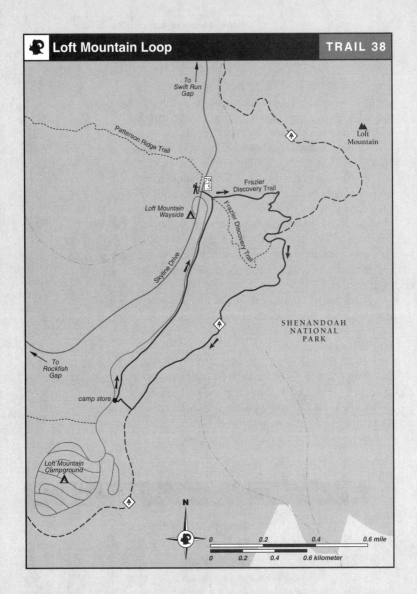

To
Swift Run
Gap

Patterson Ridge Trail

Loft
Mountain

79
.5

Frazier
Discovery Trail

Loft Mountain
Wayside

Frazier Discovery Trail

Skyline Drive

SHENANDOAH
NATIONAL
PARK

To
Rockfish
Gap

camp store

Loft Mountain
Campground

N

0   0.2   0.4   0.6 mile

0   0.2   0.4   0.6 kilometer

Loft Mountain Loop

This loop is ideal for a family hike or an afternoon stroll. Start at the Loft Mountain Wayside, and take the Frazier Discovery Trail to a massive rock outcrop with an extensive view, where Loft Mountain opens to the heavens above and the lands below. Beyond the vista, pick up the world's most famous footpath, the Appalachian Trail (AT), southward through a transitional forest to meet a paved path near the Loft Mountain Campground camp store. Gently descend back to Loft Mountain Wayside. The hike is accessible for almost everyone, though the first part does climb to the rock outcrop.

Best Time

This hike is best enjoyed during the summer months in the cool of the high forest. Also that is when the Loft Mountain Wayside (camp store) and Loft Mountain Campground are open. However, the vistas from atop Loft Mountain may be hazy then. Spring and fall are better for views. Winter presents extensive views and isolation.

Finding the Trail

Loft Mountain Wayside is located at milepost 79.5, on the west side of Skyline Drive. It is 26.1 miles north of Rockfish Gap Entrance Station. The Frazier Discovery Trail leaves from the wayside near the entrance to Loft Mountain Campground.

TRAIL USE
Dayhiking,
Pets Prohibited

LENGTH
2.9 miles, 2–3 hours

CUMULATIVE
ELEVATION +/-
+450'/-450'

DIFFICULTY
– 1 **2** 3 4 5 +

TRAIL TYPE
Loop

START & FINISH
N38° 15.771'
W78° 39.634'

FEATURES
Ridgeline
Autumn Colors
Wildflowers
Geologic Interest
Great Views

FACILITIES
Restrooms
Water
Picnic tables
Wayside store
Camp store
Campground

Trail Description

 Wildflowers

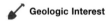 **Geologic Interest**

Leave the Loft Mountain Wayside, ▶1 and cross
Skyline Drive. Begin ascending a paved path, which
is as much gravel and moss as pavement. Shortly
intersect the Frazier Discovery Trail, turning left.
You can purchase an interpretive booklet, adding
to your hike. The dirt path splits; stay left again,
and head uphill on a rocky slope shaded with hardwoods. Before 1999, this trail was known as the
"Deadening Trail," for the settlers' practice of gir-
dling trees to kill them so that they could farm the
land beneath the standing dead trees. It doesn't have
quite the same ring as does Frazier Discovery Trail,
which is named for the family that owned much
of the area land, as well as a family that lived just
below where Loft Mountain Wayside stands today.
At 0.4 mile, curve beneath a big rock overhang on a
rocky tread. ▶2 The upthrust rock provides shelter
for storm-bound hikers.

Keep uphill amid woods to emerge onto a rock
outcrop jutting into the sky at 0.6 mile. ▶3 Enjoy this
panoramic view from 3,300 feet atop Loft Mountain.
The peaks of Shenandoah National Park poke their
heads upward to the west. Below, the Shenandoah
Valley occupies the lowlands. Massanutten Mountain
parallels the Blue Ridge upon which you stand. The

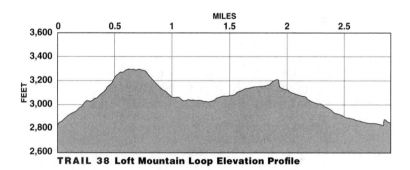

TRAIL 38 Loft Mountain Loop Elevation Profile

Alleghenies of West Virginia rise in the farthest hazy reaches. Floyd Frazier, one of the last of the Fraziers to reside in what is now the park, called this outcrop "Raven Rocks." Loft Mountain was previously known as Frazier Mountain and Lost Mountain. The outcrop is very large. Walk about, enjoying the varied vistas.

Great Views

Leave the rocky viewpoint, and join the AT, heading southbound along with the Frazier Discovery Trail. Soon, a side trail leading right opens to a second vista. ►4 Go ahead and clamber on the rocks and determine if this view is superior to the first. The outcrop is smaller, yet higher. Patterson Ridge and Big Run are to the west. Big Flat Mountain and Loft Mountain Campground are due south. From this vantage, I once saw a mother bear and two cubs strolling the leafless forest below. Ahead, stay on the AT as the Frazier Discovery Trail leaves right. Many spindly, narrow trunked trees crowd the AT. Locust and cherry trees indicate recent reforestation of pastureland where Frazier once tended cattle.

Great Views

Ridgeline

Almost the entire mountain crest here was a meadow. The cows grazed amid million-dollar views! Look for larger oak trees with widespread limbs amid the younger trees. The limbs on these older trees that once enjoyed sunlight are now denied light with reforestation, and some limbs are dying and breaking off. These older trees provided shade for the cattle when it was meadow. Parts of the trail pass through low briar-infested areas open to the sky. Keep forward on the AT beyond an overgrown road that once led 0.5 mile to the camp store. A concrete signpost still marks the intersection. The AT footbed becomes grassy beneath scraggly forest.

At 1.8 miles, turn right on a narrow trail leading 75 yards to the Loft Mountain camp store. ►5 This turn is marked with a concrete signpost. Pass behind the camp store. Take advantage of its offerings if you are hungry or thirsty. Trailside stores are rare. Just past the store, turn right onto an unnamed paved trail. Gently descend on the crumbly path beneath hawthorn and locust trees, trees that typically reclaim old fields. Look left of the trail for a water fountain made to appear as if the spigot is coming directly from the rock. Trailside fountains are about as rare as trailside camp stores. Shortly pass the Frazier Discovery Trail a final time before reaching Loft Mountain Wayside at 2.9 miles, ending your loop. ▶6

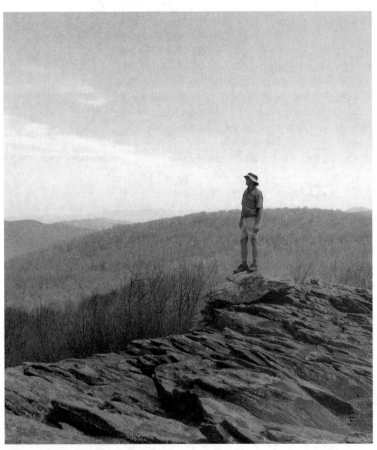

Loft Mountain *provides an early spring panorama.*

🚶 MILESTONES

►1   0.0   Loft Mountain Wayside at milepost 79.5
►2   0.4   Huge rock overhang
►3   0.6   Great views from large outcrop atop Loft Mountain
►4   0.7   Second vista, and join AT, southbound
►5   1.8   Right at spur to camp store; pick up southbound paved track
►6   2.9   Loft Mountain Wayside

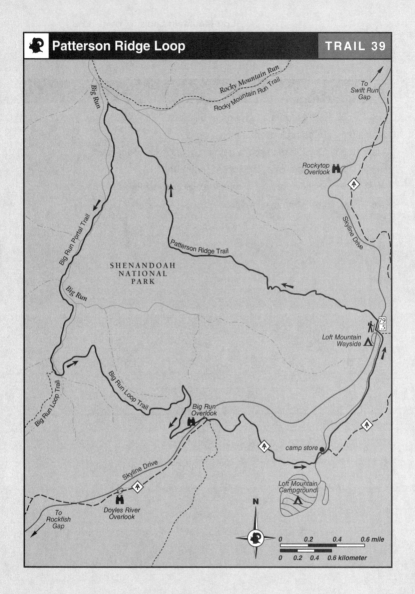

Patterson Ridge Loop — TRAIL 39

Big Run

Rocky Mountain Run

Rocky Mountain Run Trail

To Swift Run Gap

Rockytop Overlook

Skyline Drive

Patterson Ridge Trail

Big Run Portal Trail

SHENANDOAH NATIONAL PARK

Big Run

79
5

Loft Mountain Wayside

Big Run Loop Trail

Big Run Loop Trail

Big Run Overlook

camp store

Skyline Drive

Loft Mountain Campground

To Rockfish Gap

Doyles River Overlook

N

0   0.2   0.4   0.6 mile

0   0.2 0.4   0.6 kilometer

Patterson Ridge Loop

This tough loop combines a remote wilderness trail, the park's biggest stream, some high country, and a campground. Start your hike on the seldom-trod Patterson Ridge Trail, rolling west along a ridge offering some views, then pass through a striking chestnut oak forest. Descend to Big Run, literally the biggest stream in the park. Turn up Big Run, rock-hopping your way along the watercourse, with its rich forest and rock walls to reach the Big Run Loop Trail, which leads to Skyline Drive.

Cross the drive, and join the fabled Appalachian Trail (AT), heading northbound. Come near Loft Mountain Campground. End the hike by descending past the Loft Mountain camp store. The difficulty in this hike is based on the distance combined with elevation change, which amounts to a 1,500-foot drop, a 1,900-foot rise, and a final 400-foot descent back to the trailhead.

Best Time

This hike is best enjoyed from late spring through late fall. The crossings of Big Run are manageable then, and the trailhead facilities at Loft Mountain Wayside are open.

Finding the Trail

Loft Mountain Wayside is located at mile 79.5, on the west side of Skyline Drive. It is 26.1 miles north of Rockfish Gap Entrance Station. The Patterson Ridge Trail starts on the west side of Skyline Drive a little north of the Loft Mountain Wayside.

TRAIL USE
Dayhiking, Backpacking
LENGTH
9.7 miles, 5½–7 hours
CUMULATIVE ELEVATION +/-
-1,900'/+1,900'
DIFFICULTY
– 1 2 3 4 **5** +
TRAIL TYPE
Loop
START & FINISH
N38° 15.771'
W78° 39.634'

FEATURES
Ridgeline
Stream
Autumn Colors
Wildflowers
Secluded
Swimming
Great Views

FACILITIES
Restrooms
Water
Picnic tables
Wayside store
Camp store
Campground

Trail Description

Start the hike by leaving Loft Mountain Wayside ▶1 and walking northbound along Skyline Drive for approximately 50 yards. Pass the sign indicating Loft Mountain Wayside for oncoming motorists, then look left for the concrete post indicating the Patterson Ridge Trail. Turn left here (a fire road is across from you), and begin ascending a grassy track, to soon level out in hickory-oak woods. The westerly walking is easy on the well-groomed yet lightly used path. Begin a steady but gradual descent, making the first of many switchbacks at 0.6 mile. Occasional views break in partially canopied areas, rife with sumac and locust.

At 1.0 mile, a view opens on a switchback. ▶2 Here, you can gander northwest through the Big Run Portal to Massanutten Mountain, the Shenandoah Valley, and the rock outcrops and talus slopes of the lower Big Run Valley. The well-groomed single-track trail hastens downward only to meet a gap at 1.1 miles and then climb. The ascent eases as the Patterson Ridge Trail slips over to the northeast side of the ridge. Obscured views of Rocky Mountain and Rocky Mountain Run open. The path levels out for some distance in gnarled oaks and wind-sculpted pines before making a last

 Ridgeline

Great Views

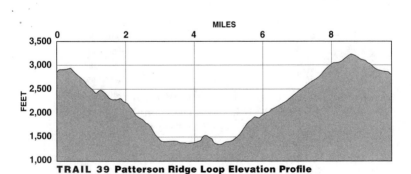

TRAIL 39 Patterson Ridge Loop Elevation Profile

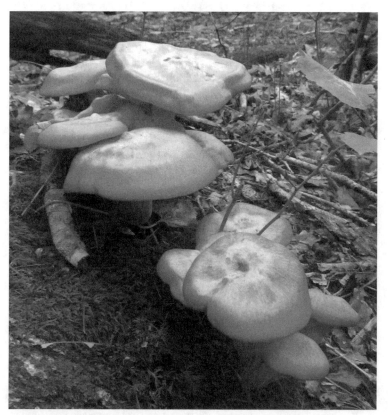

Wonders at Shenandoah *come in packages big and small, such as these woodland mushrooms.*

climb to a knob. Here, at 1.9 miles, the trail curves north onto the dividing ridge between Big Run and Rocky Mountain Run. Keep descending on the nose of this ridge, passing through a striking forest of gray-trunked chestnut oaks.

Autumn Colors

The downhill accelerates. Be glad you aren't going up this. The woods thicken after passing through a wooded talus slope. Reach the Big Run Portal Trail and the low point of the hike at 3.2 miles. ▶3 Turn left here, heading up the Big Run

Stream

 Wildflowers

Swimming

**Your efforts will be
well-rewarded on
this circuit.**

Great Views

Ridgeline

Portal Trail. Big Run flows off to your right. Trace an old fire road through plush woods where white pines and white oaks prevail. The ascent is negligible as you hike the wide valley. Intermittent wet weather tributaries cross the path. Watch for rock outcrops bordering Big Run. Rock-hop Big Run at 3.8 miles, as a rock bluff forces the trail to the right bank. Cross the stream again at 4.1 miles, just below a big pool where trout can be seen. A third crossing at 4.3 miles takes you back to the right bank, still ascending in woods dominated by tall white pines. The ascent picks up as you step over a tributary coming in from your right.

At 4.7 miles, you curve south, up a tributary into a cove hardwood forest, where tulip trees rise regal and gray. Reach the Big Run Loop Trail at 5.2 miles. ►4 Stay left here, as the Big Run Loop Trail passes an area where camping is prohibited and crosses the tributary you've been following. Watch for an overhanging rock shelter just beyond this crossing. Leave the sound of water behind while climbing into pine-oak-laurel woods on a slim mountainside path.

Crest out on a ridge dividing branches of Big Run at 5.6 miles. Gain views of the mountain crest on a short descent. Keep working for the high country, passing a streamlet. Crest out again at 6.7 miles, then make two wide, loping switchbacks, now aiming for Skyline Drive. Reach a signboard just before making the Big Run Overlook at 7.4 miles. ►5 This overlook accessible by automobile presents palpable panoramas into Big Run. Keep north on Skyline Drive for 60 yards, reaching the Doyles Run parking area on the far side of the road.

Join the Doyles Run Trail and walk a few feet before meeting the AT. Turn left here, northbound on the AT, amid locust trees, cherry trees, and thick underbrush. Much of the area is open overhead. Keep a slight ascent. Look for occasional large oak trees with widespread limbs, indicating the former openness of the regenerating forest. Level out at 7.9 miles, reach an outcrop, with north and west views to Brown Mountain and Big Run watershed. ►6 The path gently climbs, surmounting the 3,000-foot mark.

 Great Views

Meet a spur trail leading to the Loft Mountain camp store at 8.4 miles. ►7 Stay left with the spur, as the AT leaves right, circling Big Flat Mountain. An uptick leads to a high point and the Loft Mountain Campground amphitheater at 8.6 miles. ►8 You are entering the greater Loft Mountain developed area.

From the amphitheater, stay left downhill on a crumbly asphalt track, to soon cross the Loft Mountain Campground road and reach the camp store at 8.8 miles. ►9 Continue downhill on the asphalt path, paralleling the campground road. An easy decline leads you past the Frazier Discovery Trail to the Loft Mountain Wayside and the hike's end at 9.7 miles. ►10

⋏	**MILESTONES**	
►1	0.0	Loft Mountain Wayside at milepost 79.5
►2	1.0	View
►3	3.2	Left on Big Run Portal Trail
►4	5.2	Left on Big Run Portal Trail
►5	7.4	Big Run Overlook
►6	7.9	View
►7	8.4	Left on paved spur toward camp store
►8	8.6	Loft Mountain Campground amphitheater
►9	8.8	Camp store
►10	9.7	Loft Mountain Wayside at milepost 79.5

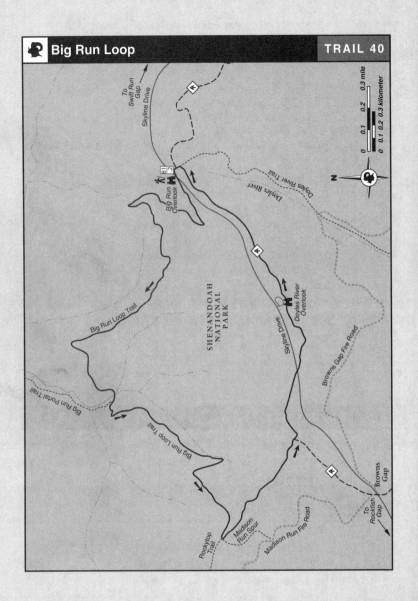

SHENANDOAH
NATIONAL
PARK

To
Swift Run
Gap
Skyline Drive

Big Run
Overlook

Doyles River Trail

Doyles River

Big Run Loop Trail

Skyline Drive

Doyles River
Overlook

Browns Gap Fire Road

Big Run Portal Trail

Big Run Loop Trail

Browns
Gap

To
Rockfish
Gap

Rockytop
Trail

Madison
Run Spur

Madison Run Fire Road

0.3 mile
0.1   0.2
0   0.1   0.2 0.3 kilometer

N

Big Run Loop

This circuit takes you through several types of forest and mountain lands. Start at Big Run Overlook, then descend into prototype oak woods. Travel a dry piney ridgeline with its attendant mountain laurel. Make your way to a tributary of Big Run, where a moist valley harbors cove hardwoods such as tulip trees. After climbing out, join a ridgeline that leads to the Appalachian Trail (AT), where you walk the spine of the Blue Ridge amid boulder fields and bluffs.

Best Time

This loop is good for spring wildflowers as it dips into the Big Run watershed. It is especially good for autumn colors since the circuit explores several forest types as it heads low and yet remains more level than not once it gets to the high country.

Finding the Trail

This hike leaves from the Big Run Overlook, on the west side of Skyline Drive at milepost 81.2. The Big Run Trail begins on the south side of the overlook.

Trail Description

Leave Big Run Overlook, ▶1 enthralling yourself with an unobstructed view of Shenandoah's biggest watershed while joining the Big Run Loop Trail. Descend the west slope of Blue Ridge on a slender single-track path. The blue-blazed trail snakes beneath sturdy oaks, striped maple, hickory, witch

TRAIL USE
Dayhiking
LENGTH
5.8 miles, 3½–4½ hours
CUMULATIVE ELEVATION +/-
-1,160'/-1,160'
DIFFICULTY
– 1 2 **3** 4 5 +
TRAIL TYPE
Loop
START & FINISH
N38° 15.224'
W78° 41.055'

FEATURES
Stream
Ridgeline
Autumn Colors
Wildflowers
Geologic Interest
Historic Interest
Great Views

FACILITIES
None

 Great Views

271

hazel, and mountain laurel. Impressive boulders are strewn about the rocky woods. At 0.2 mile, the path switchbacks right, dropping steadily. The trail briefly picks up a ridgeline before curving sharply left in a gap at 0.7 mile. Skirt around a watershed, crossing a wet weather stream at 1.2 miles. Look for a small cascade on the lower end of the crossing. Oaks, hickory, and white pine dominate the woods, along with birch, representing both moist and dry forest flora. It seems a somewhat confused forest, a mix of species. However, the variety is really indicative of the incredible biodiversity of the Appalachians, rich in ecosystems that do not delineate perfectly from one another, but rather mix and meld forest habitats. The technical term is an overlapping of ecotones.

Soon, come to a second ridgeline. This crest is cloaked in pines, coloring the pathway gold with their needles. At 1.6 miles, traverse a gap and briefly climb. Quickly, you are descending. Watery sounds sing below. Come to a perennial tributary of Big Run at 2.2 miles. ▶2 Look for the overhanging rock shelter that could come in handy during a thunderstorm on your left before reaching the stream. Rock-hop the clear and cool watercourse. Take note that it divides into tributaries just above this crossing. Tulip trees, black birch, sugar maple,

Stream

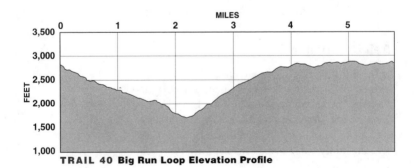

TRAIL 40 Big Run Loop Elevation Profile

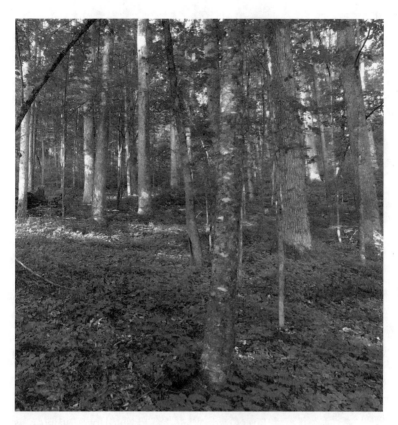

Tulip trees *rise in a cove hardwood forest.*

and other components of the cove hardwood forest predominate in this moist vale. You might want to take a break here since this is the low point of the hike and you have a substantial climb ahead. This is also your only guaranteed opportunity to get water. There once was a trail shelter in the vicinity before the area became part of the Shenandoah Wilderness and the shelter was removed.

 Wildflowers

Meet a trail junction at 2.3 miles. ▶3 To your right, the Big Run Portal Trail leaves right for the lower valley of Big Run. Stay left on the Big Run

Loop Trail, now cruising through a fern-floored forest of tulip trees. Oaks gain domain as you rise. Come along a wet-weather tributary you have been paralleling at 3.0 miles, just before turning sharply right. Continue a moderate uptick, rolling into a four-way trail junction at 3.5 miles. ▶4 The grassy gap begs a rest. That was a nearly 900-foot climb the last 1.3 miles! From here on the hike is relatively easy, with only moderate elevation changes.

Take a left at the intersection, still on the Big Run Loop Trail. This grass-lined track travels easterly and gently toward the crest of the Blue Ridge, shaded by ridgetop hickories and oaks. Pass through a section of young spindly woods rising from the fallen trunks of moth-damaged trees decades past. Your final descent bisects former pastureland, now growing up in locust. The forest ecotones keep evolving.

Meet the AT at 4.2 miles. ▶5 Turn left here, northbound, in brushy forest full of vines, fire cherry, and tulip trees. Slice through a gateway of boulders before emerging onto and crossing Skyline Drive at 4.5 miles. The trail swings over the east side of the Blue Ridge, saddling alongside some impressive gray stone bluffs. Note the rockwork on the downslope side of the AT, keeping the pathway level. At 4.8 miles, the AT emerges onto the Doyles River Overlook. ▶6 This Skyline Drive vista presents easterly looks into the Doyles River watershed, bordered by Little Flat Mountain and Cedar Mountain. The view was used by brave Confederate soldiers, who placed guns here to cover their brethren camped at nearby Browns Gap.

The trail reenters woods on the north side of the overlook. The walking remains easy on the east slope below Skyline Drive. You pass north of the Big Run Overlook and your car, but the AT keeps north to a trail junction at 5.7 miles. ▶7 Here, turn left and walk a few feet to reach the Doyles River parking area just off Skyline Drive. From this parking area,

▲ Ridgeline

Experience
Appalachian
biodiversity.

Geologic Interest

Great Views

Historic Interest

walk south a short distance along Skyline Drive to
the Big Run Overlook, completing the hike. ▶8

🚶	**MILESTONES**	
▶1	0.0	Big Run Overlook at milepost 81.2
▶2	2.2	Cross tributary of Big Run
▶3	2.3	Big Run Portal Trail leaves right
▶4	3.5	Stay left with Big Run Loop Trail at four-way junction and left again at next intersection
▶5	4.2	Left on the AT
▶6	4.8	Doyles River Overlook
▶7	5.7	Left to Doyles River parking area
▶8	5.8	Big Run Overlook at milepost 81.2

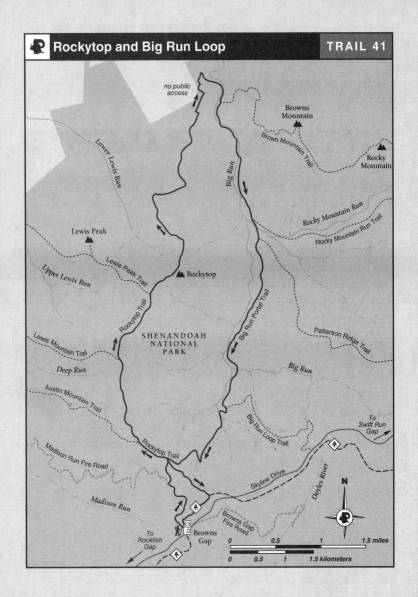

Rockytop and Big Run Loop

TRAIL 41

no public
access

Browns
Mountain

Brown Mountain Trail

Rocky
Mountain

Lower Lewis Run

Big Run

Rocky Mountain Run

Rocky Mountain Run Trail

Lewis Peak

Lewis Peak Trail

▲ Rockytop

Upper Lewis Run

Rockytop Trail

Big Run Portal Trail

Patterson Ridge Trail

SHENANDOAH
NATIONAL
PARK

Lewis Mountain Trail

Deep Run

Big Run

Austin Mountain Trail

Big Run Loop Trail

To
Swift Run
Gap

Rockytop Trail

Skyline Drive

Doyles River

Madison Run Fire Road

N

Madison Run

Browns Gap
Fire Road

83
0

Browns
Gap

To
Rockfish
Gap

0   0.5   1   1.5 miles

0   0.5   1   1.5 kilometers

Rockytop and Big Run Loop

This loop takes you along the high ridge of Rockytop Mountain where talus slopes and open boulders make for solitude-filled lookouts of the adjacent mountainscape and Shenandoah Valley beyond. Drop into crystalline Big Run, exploring the gorgeous valley of the park's largest watershed from low to high. The Big Run watershed is one of Shenandoah's backpacking destinations, even on the adjacent high ridges, where you must bring your own water.

Best Time

Since Big Run—the largest watershed in the park—has to be crossed numerous times, this circuit is best completed from late spring through late fall. Views are farthest reaching in spring and fall, but summer is best for fishing and swimming and enjoying the clear pools of Big Run.

Finding the Trail

The hike starts at the Browns Gap parking area at milepost 83.0 on Skyline Drive. From the Rockfish Gap Entrance Station, take Skyline Drive north for 21.6 miles to trailhead, on your left.

Trail Description

Leave the Browns Gap parking area, ▶1 and easily descend on Madison Run Fire Road. The Browns Gap Turnpike, built in 1805, originally laid out the modern gravel track you follow. Civil War troops crossed the Blue Ridge on the road in their

TRAIL USE
Dayhiking, Backpacking
LENGTH
13.3 miles, 8–10 hours
**CUMULATIVE
ELEVATION +/-**
-1,570'/-1,570'
DIFFICULTY
– 1 2 3 4 **5** +
TRAIL TYPE
Loop
START & FINISH
N38° 14.428'
W78° 42.654'

FEATURES
Stream
Ridgeline
Autumn Colors
Historic Interest
Great Views
Steep
Swimming
Secluded

FACILITIES
None

Historic Interest

Ridgeline

Autumn Colors

Secluded

Shenandoah Valley skirmishes. At 0.7 mile, after a sharp right turn, look for a trail marker on your right. ▶2 This is the Madison Run Spur Trail. Turn right and trace the spur uphill through pines 0.3 mile to a gap and a four-way trail junction. Turn left onto the Rockytop Trail. ▶3

The path undulates along an oak and hickory ridgetop to arrive at yet another trail junction at 1.4 miles. ▶4 Bear right, staying on the Rockytop Trail, as it slips around the east side of a knob. The trail maintains a nearly level course, presenting views of the Blue Ridge and Big Run. Come to a sag at 2.0 miles, then swing to the southwest of another knob. The vegetation morphs to pine-mountain laurel-oak woodland.

Bisect a rock field, and come to another gap. The trail then straddles the ridge while passing over a couple of small knobs. In summer wildflowers color the understory. Views open to your east of Skyline Drive just before you meet the little-used Lewis Peak Trail at 3.3 miles. ▶5 It is 1.1 miles to a worth-the-side-trip vista from Lewis Peak. Near here, wildland fires burned 1,150 acres in spring 2006. The trailside brush may still be overgrown.

This loop stays right with the Rockytop Trail. Begin descending seldom-trod track on loose stone.

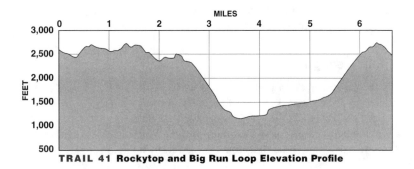

TRAIL 41 Rockytop and Big Run Loop Elevation Profile

Confront an open sun-splashed scree slope at 3.6 miles. Nearby, a knob of Rockytop rises. This unnamed knob is actually higher than the Rockytop marked on topographic maps, which is where you are at this point. Beyond that, the Shenandoah Valley stretches across the flats. The southern tip of Massanutten Mountain rises as a backdrop. Drop from the scree into a gap at 4.0 miles. Curve around the slope of what many hikers refer to as the real Rockytop. Look back on the scree slope where you were, Lewis Peak to the southwest and the Skyline Drive beyond. This Rockytop arguably offers better views than the first scree slope.

 Great Views

Enter a mix of rock and tree, the deposition of which allows more views to the west and northwest. Open onto breathtaking vistas of Shenandoah Valley at 4.7 miles while climbing away in switchbacks. Note the bigtooth aspen trees here atop the mountain. Drift through young woods and bands of scree into a gap at 5.0 miles. Blueberries grow thick amid the rock, shrubby oaks, and squat pines. At 5.3 miles, the sandy trail drops in earnest toward Big Run. Until the low-slung sporadic forest grows back fully, enjoy nearly continuous views of the Shenandoah Valley below, pinpointing field, forest, and farm. Occasional switchbacks ease the single-track's downgrade.

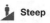 Steep

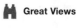 Great Views

At 6.5 miles, reach a gap. ▶6 It is only 0.2 mile to the park boundary (where there is not public access). You turn right onto the Big Run Portal Trail, overlain on an old roadbed. The easy hiking is a relief after miles of loose stones and narrow tread. Descend in hickory-oak-laurel woods to span Big Run on a wide, metal bridge at 7.0 miles. Enjoy looking at the stone slabs, pools, and gravel bars of the stream.

 Stream

Pass the Brown Mountain Trail just beyond the bridge as you hike upstream in thick woods of maple, dogwood, witch hazel, and white pine aplenty. Alder bushes, green grasses, and splotchy sycamores rise along the watercourse. Rock-hop Big Run at 7.3 miles. Look up and downstream at

 Autumn Colors

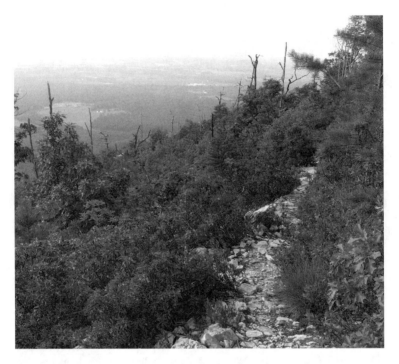

Excellent vistas open *of the Shenandoah Valley from the Rockytop Trail.*

canyon walls rising above the forest. In times of high flow, these crossings are challenging; use good sense. In summer, you will likely see more rock than water, allowing dry-shod crossings at normal water levels.

Big Run often braids around islands. Ahead, the trail follows a stony stream braid. Cross Big Run once again at 7.7 miles. The wide flats of this vale were once cultivated. Look for evidence of old homesites, including walnut trees overtaking former fields. Cross Big Run at 8.2 and 8.3 miles in succession to reach a trail junction at 8.5 miles. ▶7 Big Run and Rocky Mountain Run come together here, forming a large and relatively flat drainage basin. Continue on the Big Run Portal Trail, rock-hopping Rocky Mountain Run and walking a peninsula

Swimming

Historic Interest

between Rocky Mountain Run and Big Run. The trail gradient remains mild. Intersect the Patterson Ridge Trail at 8.7 miles. Stay on the Big Run Portal Trail under a green tunnel, crossing Big Run and its feeder streams several times.

At 10.3 miles, Big Run leaves left and the trail stays right, tracing a tributary under black birches. Meet the Big Run Loop Trail at 10.9 miles, in a lush cove of tulip trees. ►8 You have gained 500 feet the last 4 miles but now are fixing to ascend 1,100 feet in two miles. Take the fork to the right, climbing the steep trail along a slope, paralleling a tributary of Big Run. The Big Run Loop Trail switchbacks right at 11.6 miles, nearing the tributary before curving away into oak-mountain laurel woods. Reach a gap and familiar trail junction at 12.1 miles. ►9 Turn left, staying on the Big Run Loop Trail as it ascends gently on a grass-lined track. Cross a brushy knob before intersecting the Appalachian Trail (AT) at 12.8 miles. ►10 Turn right on the AT, and swing southward on an easy track. A mild downgrade in maples and oaks brings you to Browns Gap and the loop's end at 13.3 miles. ►11

 Steep

		MILESTONES
►1	0.0	Browns Gap parking area at milepost 83.0
►2	0.7	Right on Madison Run Spur Trail
►3	1.0	Left on Rockytop Trail
►4	1.4	Right to stay on Rockytop Trail
►5	3.3	Right to stay on Rockytop Trail as Lewis Peak Trail leaves left
►6	6.5	Right on Big Run Portal Trail
►7	8.5	Rocky Mountain Run Trail leaves left
►8	10.9	Right on Big Run Loop Trail
►9	12.1	Stay left on Big Run Loop Trail at gap
►10	12.8	Right, southbound, on the AT
►11	13.3	Browns Gap parking area at milepost 83.0

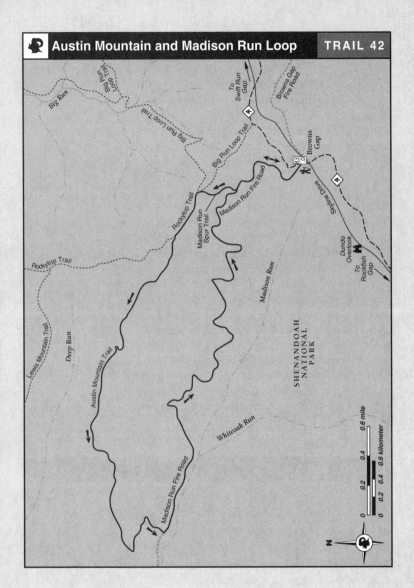

Austin Mountain and Madison Run Loop

This lesser-hiked loop has plenty of rewards. Start at historic Browns Gap, tracing a modernized toll path, then join Austin Mountain Trail. This ridge-running trek takes you past clearings and over several talus slopes that avail seldom-seen outstanding views. Descend in pines to reach the valley of Madison Run, where rich forest shades a trout stream. Rejoin the roadbed and take it up the valley, winding along ridges and hollows back to Browns Gap.

TRAIL USE
Dayhiking, Backpacking

LENGTH
8.8 miles, 5–6½ hours

CUMULATIVE ELEVATION +/-
-1,260'/+1,260'

DIFFICULTY
– 1 2 3 **4** 5 +

TRAIL TYPE
Loop

START & FINISH
N38° 14.428'
W78° 42.654'

FEATURES
Stream
Ridgeline
Autumn Colors
Wildflowers
Great Views
Historic Interest

FACILITIES
None

Best Time

Every season has something to offer on this hike. Elevations are generally low, and the hike has no fords, making it a good winter option. In summer and fall, wildflowers proliferate along Madison Run Fire Road. Enjoy views on clear days during spring and autumn.

Finding the Trail

The hike starts at the Browns Gap parking area at milepost 83.0 on Skyline Drive. From the Rockfish Gap Entrance Station, take Skyline Drive north for 21.6 miles to trailhead, on your left.

Trail Description

Leave Browns Gap beyond a chain gate, ▶1 descending gently on the Madison Run Fire Road. Many people have passed this way using what was Browns Gap Turnpike, built in 1805. Civil War troops crossed the Blue Ridge here. Since the edges of this

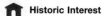

Historic Interest

Wildflowers

fire road are kept open, colorful summer and fall wildflowers, such as asters, line the way. The walking is easy on the smooth gravel track, unlike many other trails at Shenandoah National Park, and makes a good alternative for the foot-weary walker. Pines and oaks rise in the bordering woodlands, only partially shading the track. Madison Run is dropping sharply to your left. The road is used for fire management in this piney parcel of Shenandoah. Rangers also drive the track on patrol and access the western park lowlands.

Soak in seldom-seen Shenandoah vistas.

At 0.7 mile, on a sharp right turn, look for a concrete signpost on your right that marks the Madison Run Spur Trail. ▶2 Leave the gravel track for a needle-carpeted foot trail, heading uphill. The fire road will be your return route. Follow the spur 0.3 mile to a gap and a four-way trail junction. Turn left on the ridge-running Rockytop Trail. ▶3 The grass-lined path ambles west over which rise hickory, maple, oak, locust, and pin cherry.

Autumn Colors

Reach another trail junction at 1.4 miles. Bear left on the Austin Mountain Trail, making a westward track far below an unnamed knob. The south-facing slope is cloaked in pines, azaleas, and blueberries. Seclusion is yours. Usage drops off after each intersection, yet the path is well maintained, an advantage of being in Shenandoah

Ridgeline

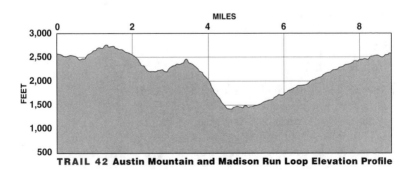

TRAIL 42 Austin Mountain and Madison Run Loop Elevation Profile

National Park. The trailbed seems quite rocky after the smooth fire road. At 1.9 miles, in blueberries, look left for views of talus-sided Blackrock, a visible rock summit, wooded Trayfoot Mountain, and Furnace Mountain.

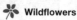 Great Views

At 2.2 miles, the trail drops sharply down the spine of a ridge and then continues through grassy woodland. Make a sharp switchback to the left, and hit a gap at 2.6 miles. Work your way along the south side of Austin Mountain on an uptick. Absorb views of the Shenandoah Valley, then gaze back at Dundo Overlook on Skyline Drive at 3.1 miles. ▶4 Reach the first of a series of talus slopes, at 3.5 miles. The high knob of Furnace Mountain stands directly across Madison Run, and the lowlands can be seen through the portal of Madison Run. Ahead, large rock outcrops also offer vista points.

Great Views

At mile 4.0, make a sharp switchback to the left. The trail drops more than 500 feet in the next half mile. Cross more talus, mixed with sporadic tree cover and join a wet-weather draw. Look for a leveled area that once housed a dismantled and forgotten structure. Cross the wet-weather draw, then intersect the Madison Run Fire Road at 4.5 miles. ▶5

Stream

Wildflowers

The fire road goes both directions. Madison Run flows on the far side of the woods. It is a crystalline stream with pools harboring brook trout. To complete the loop, head left on the fire road, wandering up the wide, wooded flat. The road rises well above the stream, allowing good looks of the water, especially when the valley tightens on this side of the creek. At 5.2 miles, the track bridges a tributary coming in from the left. A shaded grassy area lies beside the stream. Follow the tributary vale where tulip trees rise pencil straight toward the sky, along with white oaks and red maple.

Continue climbing and make a big switchback to the right. Begin a pattern of angling up mid-slope,

❀ Autumn Colors

turning into tributaries of Madison Run that will likely be dry and then curving around dry ridges dividing them. These culverted tributaries come at 5.9, 6.2, 6.6, 7.0, and 7.3 miles. Beyond here, the trail circles around a ridge and levels off at 7.5 miles, even going down for a bit. ▶6 Grab some air because the trail rises again. Complete the loop portion of the

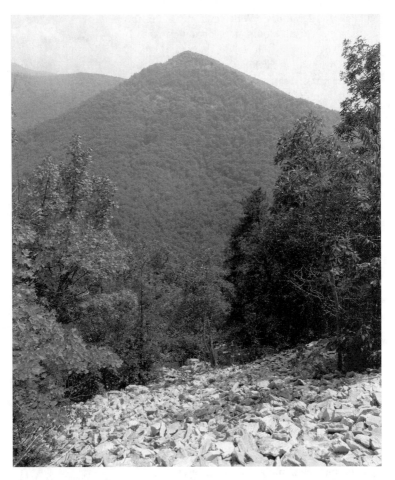

Furnace Mountain *stands proud as viewed from this Austin Mountain talus slope.*

hike at 8.1 miles. ▶7 You now have but 0.7 mile and
150 feet of climbing ahead. Return to Browns Gap at
8.8 miles, finishing the circuit. ▶8

🚶 MILESTONES

▶1	0.0	Browns Gap parking area at milepost 83.0
▶2	0.7	Right on Madison Run Spur Trail
▶3	1.0	Left on Rockytop Trail
▶4	3.1	Begin series of great views
▶5	4.5	Left on Madison Run Fire Road
▶6	7.5	Level off on ridge
▶7	8.1	Complete loop and backtrack
▶8	8.8	Browns Gap parking area at milepost 83.0

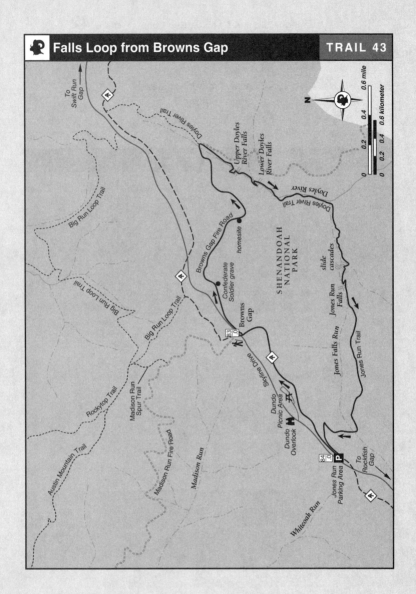

Falls Loop from Browns Gap

Water lovers will fall for this loop. The trail passes three major cataracts and numerous other cascades as it explores two boulder-strewn canyons connected by the Appalachian Trail (AT). The hike up Jones Run passes some old-growth tulip trees with impressive girths. The trail grades are generally moderate. Add a little human history, and you have a great loop hike.

Best Time

This waterfall extravaganza is best in spring. The wildflowers offer up a colorful frame for the bold cataracts you will see. Summer is nice and cool, but can be crowded, especially the Doyles River Trail. The streams will likely be low in autumn. Ice forms on the cascades during brisk winter days.

Finding the Trail

The hike starts at the Browns Gap parking area at milepost 83.0 on Skyline Drive. From the Rockfish Gap Entrance Station, take Skyline Drive north for 21.6 miles to trailhead, on your left.

Trail Description

Cross Skyline Drive ►1 and immediately begin descending on the Browns Gap Fire Road, the current name of the turnpike (Madison Run Fire Road, which leaves west from the gap near the parking area, is the western relic of this turnpike). Look for a small path leaving the road to your left at mile 0.4. ►2 Scramble

TRAIL USE
Dayhiking, Backpacking

LENGTH
7.0 miles, 4–5 hours

CUMULATIVE ELEVATION +/-
-1,280'/+1,280'

DIFFICULTY
– 1 2 3 **4** 5 +

TRAIL TYPE
Loop

START & FINISH
N38° 14.428'
W78° 42.654'

FEATURES
Stream
Ridgeline
Autumn Colors
Waterfalls
Wildflowers
Old-Growth
Geologic Interest
Historic Interest

FACILITIES
None

a few feet up this path to the grave of William H. Howard, Confederate States of America soldier. The carved stone slab marks his grave. Return to the fire road, and continue down it on a gentle grade, passing through a stand of pines. Views toward the Piedmont open through the trees.

The wide track makes for easy walking. On your left at 0.9 mile, a brushy area contains relics indicating former human habitation such as piled rocks. ▶3 Imagine the forest as cleared and cultivated. As the trail swings to the left, the canopy of trees and oaks thickens. Watch for some large trailside trees, including a noteworthy tulip tree at 1.2 miles. Cross an iron bridge spanning sassy and shallow Doyles River. Reach a trail junction at 1.7 miles. ▶4

Turn right onto Doyles River Trail. Other hikers, who have come from Skyline Drive and the upper Doyles River Trailhead, will join you. The footpath descends along lively Doyles River. Cross the waterway—an easy rock-hop—at mile 1.9. This vale was once full of hemlocks, but an invasive insect known as the woolly adelgid killed them by sucking out their sap. The woolly adelgid is thought to have been introduced to the United States from Asia in 1924. Nearly all the hemlocks in the park have succumbed to this deadly pest, save for ones the park has treated with an insecticide injected into the ground below

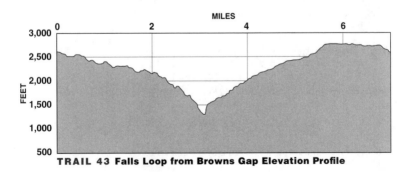

TRAIL 43 Falls Loop from Browns Gap Elevation Profile

Turnpike through Browns Gap

Browns Gap, where you start your hike, is a location of historical significance. Confederate general Stonewall Jackson passed
through here in early 1862 while outwitting Union forces in the
mountains around the Shenandoah Valley. Jackson's local knowl-
edge left the Northerners bamboozled time and again. Browns
Gap was important because of the strategic turnpike that went
through it, connecting Richmond with the Shenandoah Valley.

You walk the very same turnpike built in 1805 on the first leg
of this hike. Think of all the farmers loaded with corn (and liquid
corn, also known as moonshine), circuit-riding preachers, traveling hucksters, weary immigrants, and Civil War soldiers who
walked this way. And now you come.

the trees. Hardwoods now dominate the forest.
Wildflowers carpet the woodland floor.

Doyles River Trail continues along the watercourse but swings away as it approaches Upper
Doyles Falls. At mile 2.1 a side trail leads to the
dark pool at the base of the three-tier, 30-foot falls
that drops into a bouldery glen at the point where
a tributary feeds the river. ►5 The canyon tightens;
Doyles River makes frenzied drops. Unnamed cascades accompany you downstream until a sharp
switchback leads to the base of Lower Doyles Falls
at mile 2.4. ►6 Lower Doyles Falls is the steeper
and more spectacular of the two at 63 feet. It dives
over a rock lip and then spills in ribbons, strands,
and crashing channels over multiple tiers to finally
land in a pool before charging on. The cataract looks
different depending on the flow level. A rock wall
extends across the far gorge.

Waterfall

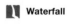
Waterfall

The trail squeezes down the narrow, very rugged
gorge, using a wooden bridge to span a cascading
tributary spilling into Doyles River at 2.7 miles. At
2.9 miles, find a deep pool between quickly moving
rapids. At 3.1 miles, in a small flat that would make
a good lunch spot, come to a trail marker and the

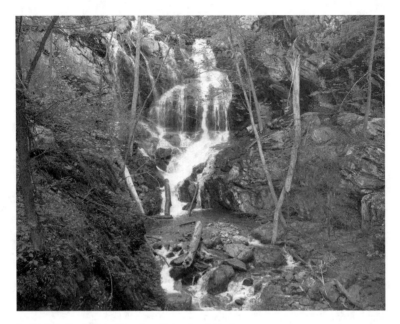

Lower Doyles Falls *crashes through a rock cathedral.*

end of Doyles River Trail. ▶7 Jones Run and Doyles River merge below the signpost. Notice the sycamores in the lower valley—the climate is just too cold for them upstream on either branch.

Veer right on lesser-used Jones Run Trail, and begin to climb, rock-hopping Jones Run at 3.3

🌲 **Old-Growth**

miles. ▶8 Impressive tulip trees grow tall with such wide diameters that it would take several hikers to encircle them. Look up the slope. Jones Run gorge is littered with huge boulders. Keep an eye on the creek too, as many scenic cascades tumble down the relentless watercourse, including some sliding cascades. At 3.8 miles, step over a tributary. ▶9 You arrive at Jones Run Falls, where water spills 45 feet over a solid rock wall. Large waterside rock slabs

🏳 **Waterfall**

make for good observation points. Feel the cool air and mist from the cataract.

The trail turns sharply left, circumventing a rock rampart. Achieve the top of the falls. The path traces Jones Run past more cascades before veering away from the creek. Gently ascend through a cove-hardwood forest with an open understory of grass and ferns. At 5.0 miles, join an old wagon road. The path widens. Step over Jones Run, minute at this point at 5.2 miles. ▶10 Leave the wagon track, also heading for Browns Gap. The Jones Run Trail ascends and makes a sharp left turn at 5.4 miles.

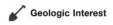 **Geologic Interest**

Meet the AT at 5.7 miles. ▶11 The Jones Run Trailhead and parking area are just steps away. Turn right on the AT, northbound, toward Dundo Picnic Area. Dry species, such as mountain laurel and chestnut oak, straddle the grade back to Browns Gap. Pass spur trails to Dundo Picnic Area at 6.3 miles. ▶12 Intermittent views of Cedar Mountain open. The AT descends before arriving at Browns Gap. Complete your loop at 7.0 miles. ▶13

▲ **Ridgeline**

🚶	**MILESTONES**	
▶1	0.0	Browns Gap parking area at milepost 83.0
▶2	0.4	Grave of Confederate soldier William H. Howard
▶3	0.9	Old homesite
▶4	1.7	Right on Doyles River Trail
▶5	2.1	Upper Doyles River Falls
▶6	2.4	Lower Doyles River Falls
▶7	3.1	Join Jones Run Trail
▶8	3.3	Cross Jones Run
▶9	3.8	Jones Run Falls
▶10	5.2	Step over Jones Run
▶11	5.7	Right on the AT
▶12	6.3	Dundo Picnic Area
▶13	7.0	Browns Gap parking area at milepost 83.0

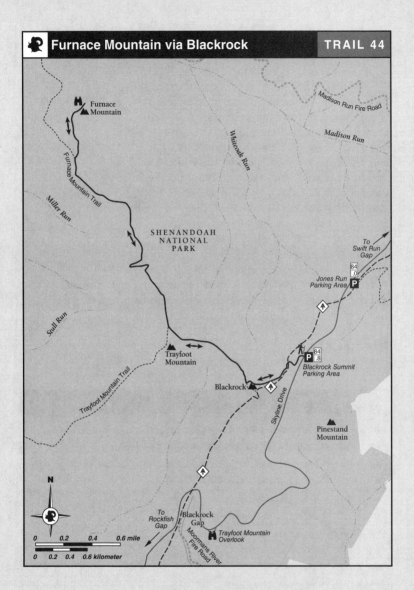

Furnace
Mountain

Madison Run Fire Road

Madison Run

Whiteoak Run

Furnace Mountain Trail

Miller Run

SHENANDOAH
NATIONAL
PARK

To
Swift Run
Gap

84
.0

Jones Run
Parking Area

Stull Run

Trayfoot
Mountain

84
.8

Blackrock Summit
Parking Area

Trayfoot Mountain Trail

Blackrock

Skyline Drive

Pinestand
Mountain

N

To
Rockfish
Gap

Blackrock
Gap

Trayfoot Mountain
Overlook

Moormans River
Fire Road

0   0.2   0.4   0.6 mile

0   0.2   0.4   0.6 kilometer

Furnace Mountain via Blackrock

This outstanding hike shows off special features of Shenandoah, namely its interesting geology that results in huge outcrops rising above the forest and open talus slopes where rocks by the thousands carpet the mountainsides. Once you finish soaking in the outstanding views of Blackrock Summit with other hikers, enter one of the park's more remote areas, availing maximum solitude. Be careful because the trail is rocky. Take your time and enjoy the solitude of Furnace Mountain.

Best Time

Take this view-laden trek when the skies are clear. You will be amply rewarded.

Finding the Trail

Blackrock parking area is at milepost 84.8 on Skyline Drive, on the west side. From Rockfish Gap Entrance Station, it is a 19.9-mile drive to the trailhead.

Trail Description

Leave the Blackrock parking area, ▶1 passing around a pole gate on the wide roadbed of the Trayfoot Mountain Trail. Locust, ferns, and grasses border the track. Begin climbing and intersect the slender, shady Appalachian Trail (AT) at 0.1 mile. ▶2 Head left, south, on the level-running master path of Shenandoah. The Trayfoot Mountain Trail runs parallel to the AT at this point and is within

TRAIL USE
Dayhiking, Backpacking

LENGTH
6.8 miles, 4–5 hours

CUMULATIVE
ELEVATION +/-
+900'/-900'

DIFFICULTY
– 1 2 **3** 4 5 +

TRAIL TYPE
Out & Back

START & FINISH
N38° 13.370'
W78° 44.010'

FEATURES
Ridgeline
Summit
Autumn Colors
Geologic Interest
Great Views
Secluded

FACILITIES
None

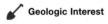 **Geologic Interest**

Great Views

Enjoy the solitude of
Furnace Mountain.

Great Views

sight. It isn't long before the woods give way and
you enter the open stones of Blackrock. ▶3 To your
left, huge boulders rise in crazy formations, making for exciting scrambling opportunities. To your
right, a gray talus slope recedes down the mountain, opening up stupendous highland panoramas.
Furnace Mountain, your destination, rises to the
west. Madison Run cuts a wooded swath between
Austin Mountain and Furnace Mountain. The valley is known as Dundo Hollow. Austin Mountain
forms a rampart to the north. More peaks rise in the
distance, while the Shenandoah Valley fades to the
horizon. This is one of the finest spots on the AT,
in my opinion.

The AT curves left to intersect the Blackrock
Spur Trail at 0.4 mile. ▶4 Turn right, joining the
spur. Make a stony passage through boulders, opening onto a rocky ridge with plentiful panoramas,
limited only by how many outcrops you want to
visit. Trailside views are numerous too. Trayfoot
Mountain stands brazen, with its talus slopes forming breaks in the forest. The valley of Paine Run
falls away to your left. This is a place to linger. Trees
eventually overtake the protuberance, and you intersect the Trayfoot Mountain Trail at 0.7 mile. ▶5

Turn right on the Trayfoot Mountain Trail,
traveling westerly on a slender ridge. Enter the

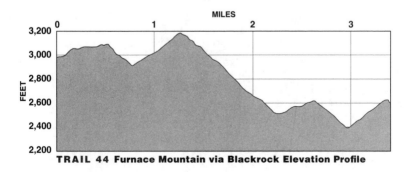
TRAIL 44 Furnace Mountain via Blackrock Elevation Profile

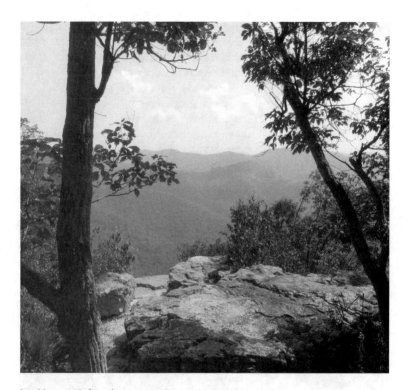

Looking north *from the outcrop at Furnace Mountain*

Shenandoah Wilderness, though you will note no difference, save for lack of other hikers. Note the lesser-used trailbed. Reach a gap, then begin climbing a grassy ridge, bordered with brushy, younger locust, sumac, and blackberries. This area was hit hard by the gypsy moth, which defoliated trees. They were introduced to the northeastern United States from Europe in 1869. The insects reached Shenandoah in 1983 and wrought havoc; their legacy still can be seen three decades later.

▲ **Ridgeline**

  Ascend to an intersection at 1.3 miles. ▶6 Here, it is but 0.2 mile to the summit of Trayfoot Mountain. You are at the high point of this hike, above 3,000 feet. Leave the Trayfoot Mountain Trail, and turn right on the Furnace Mountain Trail. I have never seen another hiker past this point. Oak halls, along with hickories and low-slung sassafras, shade the path. Drop off the northern flank of Trayfoot Mountain, and pass through a talus slope. The loose rock makes for tough footing. The trail loses elevation steadily, making two sharp turns, first to the left, then to the right. Arrive at a gap at 2.3 miles. The ridge narrows here as you cross an open forest

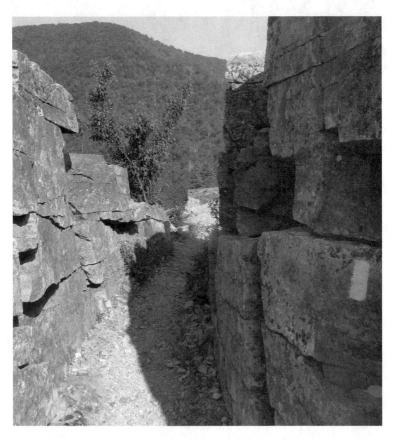

Trayfoot Mountain Trail *squeezes between stone ramparts en route to Furnace Mountain.*

Secluded

of oaks, pines, and mountain laurel. Blueberries form a ground cover and ripen in July.

Surmount a knob, then meet the side trail to Furnace Mountain summit at 3.0 miles. ▶7 Turn right on the spur trail, and begin climbing through pine-oak and laurel, mixed in with burnished quartz. As you ascend, wide views of the Shenandoah Valley open to your left. Bisect a small scree slope at 3.2 miles, then level off in a flat.

Summit

Descend slightly from the small wooded flat on the north side of Furnace Mountain to reach a distended rock outcrop. ▶8 Here, you can over-look the lower canyon of Madison Run in Dundo Hollow. Directly across the canyon stands Austin Mountain. Rockytop rises behind Austin Mountain. The main crest of the Blue Ridge stretches to your right. Relax and enjoy the view; you'll most likely have it all to yourself.

Great Views

	MILESTONES	
▶1	0.0	Blackrock parking area at milepost 84.8
▶2	0.1	Meet the AT
▶3	0.3	First-rate view from Blackrock
▶4	0.4	Blackrock Spur Trail
▶5	0.7	Trayfoot Mountain Trail
▶6	1.3	Furnace Mountain Trail
▶7	3.0	Spur to Furnace Mountain summit
▶8	3.4	Furnace Mountain summit

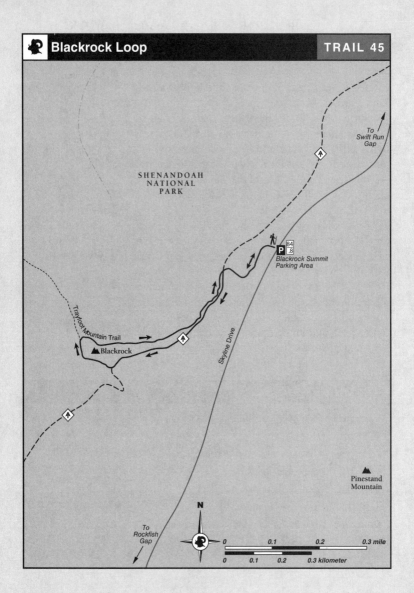

Blackrock Loop

TRAIL 45

SHENANDOAH
NATIONAL
PARK

To
Swift Run
Gap

Blackrock Summit
Parking Area

Trayfoot Mountain Trail

Blackrock

Skyline Drive

Pinestand
Mountain

N

To
Rockfish
Gap

0   0.1   0.2   0.3 mile

0   0.1   0.2   0.3 kilometer

Blackrock Loop

Shenandoah is known for its overlooks and vistas. Many can be accessed from Skyline Drive. But, as hikers know, the best views are earned on foot. Not everyone can tramp for miles to an overlook. However, this short loop around the summit of Blackrock is doable by just about everyone from 4 to 84.

Start at nearly 3,000 feet, then make your way up the Trayfoot Mountain Trail on a wide track, topping a hill. Meet the Appalachian Trail (AT) and follow it northbound. Open onto an incredible rock jumble. Views extend for miles in multiple directions. Kids enjoy scrambling over massive boulders to reach the summit of Blackrock. Adults can stay on the AT. After gaining views from several spots, reenter woods, working your way back to the trailhead.

Best Time

This child-friendly highland walk is best whenever the skies are clear, whether it is winter, spring, or fall. Summer is often hazy, yet has its share of clear days. Also, the optional rock scrambling atop Blackrock is safest when the terrain is dry.

Finding the Trail

Blackrock parking area is at milepost 84.8 on Skyline Drive, on the west side. From Rockfish Gap Entrance Station, it is a 19.9-mile drive to the trailhead.

Trail Description

A large sign at the hike's beginning ►1 details the tightly woven trail network lacing the crest of Blackrock. You

TRAIL USE
Dayhiking,
Child-Friendly

LENGTH
1.1 miles, 1–1½ hours

**CUMULATIVE
ELEVATION +/-**
+165'/-165'

DIFFICULTY
– **1** 2 3 4 5 +

TRAIL TYPE
Loop

START & FINISH
N38° 13.370'
W78° 44.010'

FEATURES
Summit
Ridgeline
Autumn Colors
Great Views
Geologic Interest

FACILITIES
None

Autumn Colors

Ridgeline

Geologic Interest

Great Views

walk under a mixed canopy of locust and other hardwoods. The large flowering black cohosh exhibits its fragrant white cylindrical flowers in midsummer. To the left of the trail brushy woods proliferate. Look for blackened trunks of trees from a past fire. Curve uphill then come to the AT at 0.1 mile. ▶2 A few short steps connect the AT to the Trayfoot Mountain Trail here. For now, stay straight on the wide Trayfoot Mountain Trail, resuming an uptick, topping out at 0.3 mile. A hill rises yet higher to your left. Observe how the trail was used as a fire line. To the left, you can see old blackened trunks amid the regrowth, whereas to the right of the trail the woods exhibit no signs of burn within the past decade.

The slope opens to your left. Blackberries attract man and beast alike. At 0.5 mile, come to a four-way intersection. ▶3 Here, you meet the AT yet again. Another map displays the trail system here. Turn right, northbound, on the AT. Soon you open onto the south side of the rock jumble that is Blackrock.

Hundreds, perhaps thousands of broken stones rise in a pile prescribed by the hands of God. Views open to your south, then west. Paine Hollow creates a void below, while the forest and rock slopes of Trayfoot Mountain rise in the distance. The boulder stack of Blackrock rises to your right, coming

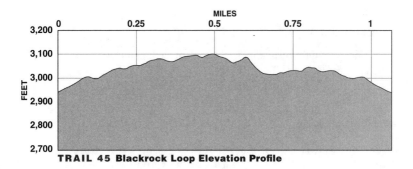

TRAIL 45 Blackrock Loop Elevation Profile

together in a crown above. The stones of Blackrock are grayish, but a dark lichen known as rock tripe grows on them, giving them a dark appearance from afar. It will be hard to keep active kids from scaling the boulders. Maybe you should join them. The view spreads 270 degrees from the top!

 Summit

Intersect the Blackrock Spur Trail at 0.6 mile. ▶4 More interesting geological formations, including mammoth boulder "gates" through which you walk, are down that trail. This loop stays with the AT as it continues circling Blackrock. A more accessible rock outcrop—as opposed to the jumble above you—stretches left toward Trayfoot Mountain.

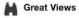

Fantastic vistas from rock outcrops await kids from 9 to 90.

And as you turn north, a talus slope falls hundreds of feet down the mountain, revealing a wealth of national park beyond. Furnace Mountain forms a knob to the west. The talus slope drops to Madison Run below; the valley is also called Dundo Hollow. Austin Mountain constructs a wooded wall across Madison Run. More Shenandoah highlands meld into the horizon, while the Shenandoah Valley flanks the lowlands below. Pull up a boulder and soak in the vista.

Great Views

Leave the open rock expanse for the shady single-track fern-bordered AT. The walking is easy and level. It isn't long before you meet the short spur to the wide Trayfoot Mountain Trail and complete your loop. From there, backtrack to the parking lot, completing the walk. ▶5

	MILESTONES	
▶1	0.0	Blackrock parking area at milepost 84.8
▶2	0.1	Pass the AT
▶3	0.5	Right on the AT
▶4	0.6	Blackrock Spur Trail leaves left
▶5	1.1	Blackrock parking area at milepost 84.8

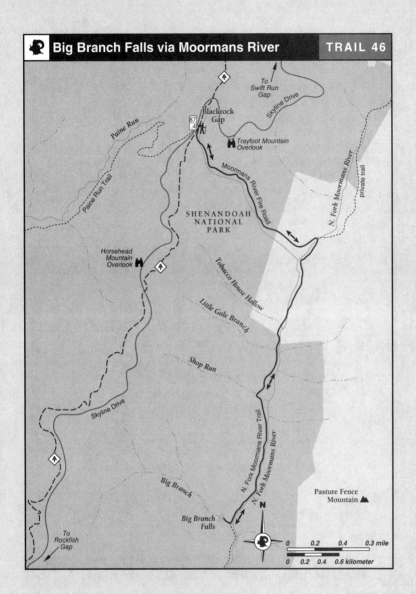

Big Branch Falls via Moormans River   TRAIL 46

To Swift Run Gap

Skyline Drive

Paine Run

Blackrock Gap

87

Trayfoot Mountain Overlook

Moormans River Fire Road

SHENANDOAH NATIONAL PARK

N. Fork Moormans River

private trail

Paine Run Trail

Horsehead Mountain Overlook

Tobacco House Hollow

Little Gale Branch

Shop Run

Skyline Drive

Big Branch

N. Fork Moormans River Trail

N. Fork Moormans River

To Rockfish Gap

Big Branch Falls

Pasture Fence Mountain ▲

N

0   0.2   0.4   0.3 mile

0   0.2   0.4   0.6 kilometer

Big Branch Falls via Moormans River

This is perhaps the most bypassed, ignored, and undervisited trail-accessible waterfall in all of Shenandoah National Park. Enjoy the seclusion. Start on Skyline Drive, and descend to the North Fork Moormans River. Cruise along the scenic stream with cascades and pools in a deep valley bordered by high ridges. Everywhere-you-look beauty overlays this gorge bordered by Pasture Fence Mountain on one side and the Blue Ridge on the other. Finally, climb along low-flowing Big Branch, with its open watery bowls divided by rock slabs where the stream flows in slide cascades.

Best Time

Big Branch Falls are their best when the water is up, but since you must cross North Fork Moormans River, you don't want the water too high. Therefore, mid-spring through midsummer is best.

Finding the Trail

The Moormans River Fire Road begins at Blackrock Gap at milepost 87.4 on Skyline Drive.

Trail Description

Your hike leaves Blackrock Gap, elevation 2,330 feet, ▶1 to moderately descend on the Moormans River Fire Road. The Appalachian Trail (AT) is just to your right. At 0.1 mile, step over a small branch that the trail begins to parallel.

TRAIL USE
Dayhiking, Backpacking

LENGTH
7.6 miles, 5–6 hours

CUMULATIVE ELEVATION +/-
-880'/+880'

DIFFICULTY
– 1 2 3 **4** 5 +

TRAIL TYPE
Out & Back

START & FINISH
N38° 12.395'
W78° 44.973'

FEATURES
Stream
Autumn Colors
Wildflowers
Waterfall
Swimming
Secluded

FACILITIES
None

🚶 **Secluded**

Pass through pine, black gum, oak, and hickory woodland with an understory of mountain laurel, descending gently on the wide double-track. The branch you crossed drops steeply for North Fork Moormans River.

At 1.1 miles, come to a gate on the road; you are leaving the park for a period. ▶2 The trail stays on a right-of-way, descending to a junction at 1.4 miles. Turn right and immediately cross the North Fork Moormans River on rocks. ▶3 At higher flows this crossing may be a ford. The trail follows the river downstream. Look for ironwood and black birch in this deep vale. Wildflowers color the trailside in spring. At 1.6 miles, when a private road splits left, you stay right, passing a ramshackle hunter's camp on your left. Look for the smooth gray trunks of the many beech trees that grow in the area. Their nuts are a favored wildlife food source.

Make another rock-hop of the river at 2.0 miles. ▶4 You stay on the west bank for the remainder of the hike. Bisect a small grassy clearing. Reenter the park at the crossing of Little Gale Branch at 2.1 miles. ▶5 The road takes on a more overgrown appearance and is now called the North Fork Moormans River Trail. Tightly growing, spindly trees are rising from what once

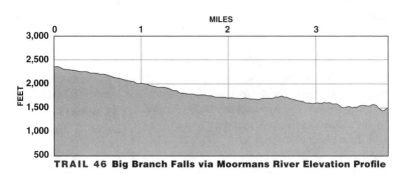

TRAIL 46 Big Branch Falls via Moormans River Elevation Profile

was barren soil, remnants of a cataclysmic flood back in the 1990s. I saw this valley then, and the reforestation is truly amazing.

Cross Shop Run at 2.3 miles. The metal remnants of an old bridge lie in state here. Before the 1995 flood Shenandoah National Park maintained this trail as a fire road. Step over an unnamed perennial stream at 2.7 miles. Come back along North Fork Moormans River at 2.9 miles. Tulip trees and sycamores rise from the streamside. Even a few hemlocks are hanging on. Gigantic boulders, gravel bars, speedy shoals, and quiet pools, some deep enough for a dip, all intermingle below. Streamside open rock slabs beckon a visit. Brook trout, rock bass, and smallmouth bass ply the waters.

Come to Big Branch at 3.7 miles. ▶6 You can see the lower drops of Big Branch Falls from the main trail. Step over the stream, then take the 0.1-mile side trail that leads right to the falls. This canyon was gouged back in '95, exposing the rock bed of the creek, making the entire scene more dramatic. The low-volume cataract drops 30 feet into a plunge pool, then another cascade slides into a second pool. Still another drop, the lowermost, dips into the deepest pool. As you explore the falls, ▶7 avoid slick spots on the open rock slabs adjacent to the moving water.

You will likely have this falls to yourself.

Swimming

Stream

Waterfall

🚶		MILESTONES
▶1	0.0	Blackrock Gap parking area at milepost 87.4
▶2	1.1	Leave park at a gate
▶3	1.4	Cross North Fork Moormans River
▶4	2.0	Cross North Fork Moormans River
▶5	2.1	Reenter park
▶6	3.7	Cross Big Branch
▶7	3.8	Big Branch Falls

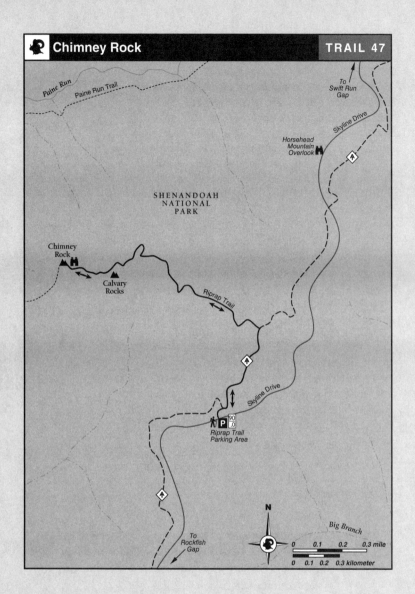

Paine Run

Paine Run Trail

To Swift Run Gap

Skyline Drive

Horsehead Mountain Overlook

SHENANDOAH NATIONAL PARK

Chimney Rock

Calvary Rocks

Riprap Trail

Skyline Drive

90
0

Riprap Trail Parking Area

To Rockfish Gap

N

Big Branch

0   0.1   0.2   0.3 mile

0   0.1   0.2   0.3 kilometer

Chimney Rock

Be careful when you get to Chimney Rock. A deep crevasse separates the actual Chimney Rock and the rock you can reach safely. At one time a short bridge spanned this crevasse, but only the metal anchors remain. The bridge was removed when the Shenandoah Wilderness was created. This wilderness adds a layer of extra protection to large disjunct tracts of land within the park.

Since the bridge to the Chimney Rock was not part of the natural landscape, it was removed. However, the views are still stellar from the outcrop adjoining Chimney Rock, as well as a point along the route to Chimney Rock.

Best Time

This hike is a winner any time of year—the exposed quartz is interesting close-up. But the views from the outcrops are at their finest in spring, fall, and on clear winter days.

Finding the Trail

The Riprap Trail parking area is located at milepost 90.0 on the west side of Skyline Drive, 14.6 miles north of the Rockfish Gap Entrance Station.

Trail Description

The hike starts on the Riprap Trail. Leave the Riprap parking area, ▶1 and walk a grand total of 83 feet before intersecting the Appalachian Trail (AT). Turn right on the AT, northbound, and climb north

---

TRAIL USE
Dayhiking, Backpacking

LENGTH
3.2 miles, 2–3 hours

CUMULATIVE
ELEVATION +/-
+480'/-480'

DIFFICULTY
– 1 **2** 3 4 5 +

TRAIL TYPE
Out & Back

START & FINISH
N38° 10.665'
W78° 45.908'

FEATURES
Ridgeline
Autumn Colors
Geologic Interest
Great Views

FACILITIES
None

Autumn Colors

Ridgeline

Great Views

through a pine-oak forest with a thick understory of azaleas, serviceberries, and mountain laurel. The evergreen mountain laurel shrubs display their pink blooms in May and June. The AT is in excellent shape here, despite the stony terrain.

Intersect the continuation of the blue-blazed Riprap Trail at 0.4 mile. ►2 Turn left as the Riprap Trail makes a sharp switchback to the right at 0.5 mile, then begin to descend, passing through a chestnut oak forest. A chestnut oak has thick leaves with wavy, rounded lobes on both sides of the leaf. Its acorns have been a primary food source for park animals since the demise of the chestnut tree in the early 1900s. Notice also a primary understory tree of the chestnut oak forest, the striped maple. The small tree is distinguished by its vertically striped bark and large goose foot–shaped leaves.

The Riprap Trail dips to a gap at 1.0 mile ►3 and begins to climb, entering a rock field. Imagine the work involved in clearing the trail here and making it more foot-friendly. Achieve the crest of the ridge at 1.2 miles. ►4 Immediately to your right is an outcrop with fine views into Paine Run below and the Shenandoah Valley beyond. Note the white quartz and the fascinating striations within. An old gnarled pine tree by the trail offers substantial shade for the hot hiker.

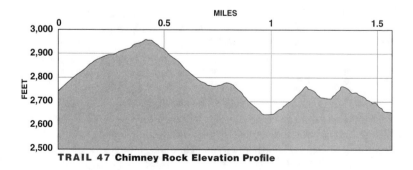

TRAIL 47 Chimney Rock Elevation Profile

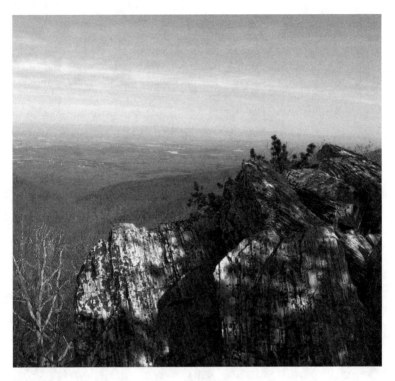

The Shenandoah Valley *stretches west as far as the clarity of the sky allows.*

Continue heading west on the narrow ridge past a series of boulders. This is all part of aptly named Rocks Mountain. You reach the Calvary Rocks, a high knob on Rocks Mountain, at 1.4 miles. ▶5 Look for an old trail leading left to the top of the Calvary Rocks. The forest has reclaimed this outcrop, which offered views in days gone by. The park service used to cut back the vegetation as they do at Skyline Drive overlooks, but they stopped the practice after the area was designated a wilderness. Pass another lichen-covered boulder field. Look for ferns hiding in the moist, shady crevasses. Descend and then take the side trail leading right to Chimney

Geologic Interest

Great Views

Rock at mile 1.7. ►6 A few steps later, emerge on a prominent quartz outcrop.

Carefully step out. No matter the season, you can find the perfect combination of sun and shade to suit the temperatures. Look below into the crevasse formerly spanned by a bridge. Now look out from left to right. First you can see the patchwork quilt of land that is the Shenandoah Valley and, beyond, the Alleghenies. Below, Paine Run cuts its way west to the South River, a tributary of the South Fork Shenandoah River. Trayfoot Mountain rises across Paine Run, which at 3,374 feet is the second highest peak in Shenandoah's South District. Open, gray talus slopes tattoo the mountainside. Finally, to your right the Blue Ridge rises majestically. There is plenty to see from here, even without a bridge to Chimney Rock.

🚶 MILESTONES

►1	0.0	Riprap Trail parking area at milepost 90.0
►2	0.4	Riprap Trail leaves left from the AT
►3	1.0	Gap
►4	1.2	Vista
►5	1.4	Old trail to Calvary Rocks
►6	1.7	Chimney Rock

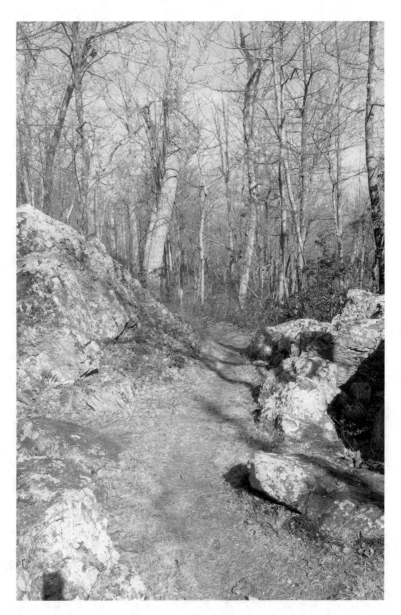

The sun *shines weakly on the Riprap Trail and adjacent embedded boulders.*

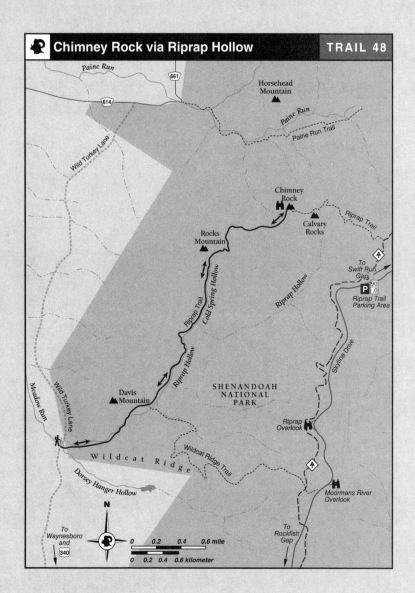

Chimney Rock via Riprap Hollow

Bring your camera with you on this hike. As you make your way up Riprap Hollow, the environment goes through dramatic changes. Start out in a lush streamside forest, pass through a narrow canyon to a deep swimming hole, open onto a piney, rocky hillside, and finally emerge onto Rocks Mountain with views from its airy, quartz outcrops.

Best Time

Spring presents plenty of wildflowers in Riprap Hollow. Summer is favorable for swimming, while fall and winter have the best views from Chimney Rock.

Finding the Trail

From the junction of US 250 and US 340 in Waynesboro, east of the South River (near Rockfish Gap), take US 340 north for 6.3 miles to VA 612, Crimora Mine Road. Turn right on VA 612, and follow it for 1.7 miles to Black Bear Lane.

Turn left and follow Black Bear Lane a short distance to Wild Turkey Lane. You will see a Shenandoah National Park post here. Veer left on Wild Turkey Lane, coming to a road split at 1.0 mile and another concrete post. You can park here, near the post, or turn right and cross a rocky streambed to reach the main parking area on the far side of the streambed. This streambed crossing can be rough for some cars.

TRAIL USE
Dayhiking

LENGTH
6.8 miles, 3½–5 hours

CUMULATIVE ELEVATION +/-
+1,210'/-1,210'

DIFFICULTY
– 1 2 3 **4** 5 +

TRAIL TYPE
Out & Back

START & FINISH
N38° 9.495'
W78° 48.721'

FEATURES
Stream
Ridgeline
Waterfall
Wildflowers
Autumn Colors
Swimming
Great Views

FACILITIES
None

Trail Description

Leave the lower parking area, ►1 cross a side stream flowing out of Dorsey Hanger Hollow, and then come to the park boundary, a trail marker, and the upper parking area. Continue straight on a rocky roadbed that enters an eye-catching forest of gum, hickory, sassafras, oaks, and pine. Mountain laurel rises from the forest floor. Occasional preserved hemlocks spread evergreen. Meadow Run gurgles off to your left. Riprap Hollow closes. At 0.6 mile the nearly level but rocky trail crosses Meadow Run.

At 0.9 mile, come to the Wildcat Ridge Trail junction. ►2 It leaves right for Skyline Drive. Continue straight on the Riprap Trail. After passing a boulder field to your left, the canyon narrows and the trail passes close to the stream. Here you may see Catawba rhododendron, rare in these parts, display its pink plumage around the beginning of June. Step over Meadow Run at 1.4 miles, ►3 then come to the Riprap Hollow swimming hole. Meadow Run makes a short slide over a stone slab and then forms a deep pool, luring in hot and sweaty hikers. A set of rock steps leads to the pool. Long ago a trail shelter was located hereabouts.

At 1.6 miles, the trail crosses Meadow Run again and climbs. At this point, the path was rerouted out

Autumn Colors

Stream

Wildflowers

Swimming

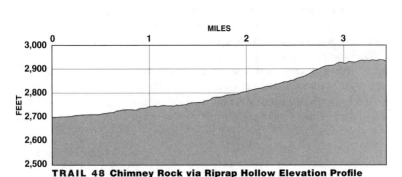

TRAIL 48 Chimney Rock via Riprap Hollow Elevation Profile

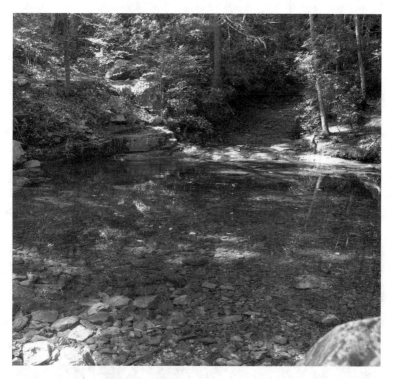

Swimming hole *in Riprap Hollow*

of the now-tight ravine for safety's sake. Enter an
open area of rock and pine. From an outcrop, gaze
down the hollow.

 Great Views

Descend back into the constricted canyon
where Meadow Run flows betwixt vertical rock
walls. Look for a series of cataracts plunging out
from the narrowest section of the canyon. ▶4
Also, look for embedded wood beams in the water
between the tightest chasm walls. These are perhaps remnants of an old dam from pre-park days.
The canyon opens, and you veer left into wooded
Cold Spring Hollow at mile 1.8. Black birches find
a home in this vale, which becomes wide, shallow,
and boulder-strewn on its upper end.

 Waterfall

▲ Ridgeline

M Great Views

The trail climbs ever more abruptly, switchbacking left into xeric pine-oak woods as it joins Rocks Mountain. Look left for views back down Meadow Run and beyond. Crest out on Rocks Mountain at 2.8 miles. ▶5 The climb is essentially over. Enjoy looks into Paine Run valley and at Trayfoot Mountain beyond. An outcrop left of the trail at 3.0 miles provides clear looks down the Paine Run portal and into Shenandoah Valley. ▶6 To your right, along the ridge, white Chimney Rock pokes out above the trees, living up to its name. Continue the cruise in scraggly burn-prone forest, coming to a side trail at mile 3.4. ▶7 Walk a few feet left and you are at Chimney Rock.

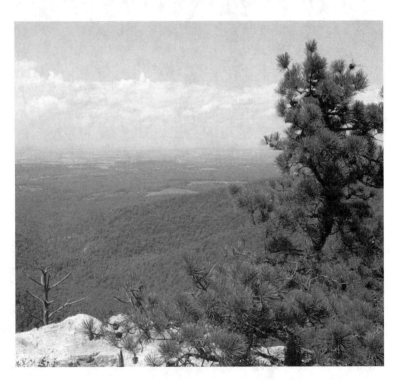

Looking down *on Paine Run and the Shenandoah Valley beyond from Rocks Mountain*

An expanse of Old Dominion grandeur opens before you. Below, Paine Run and its tributaries form veins running beneath tree-clad highlands. The massive mountain pocked with gray scree slopes is Trayfoot Mountain. The Blue Ridge stands proud to the right of Trayfoot. The Alleghenies form a rampart on the far side of the patchwork quilt of farm, field, forest road, and river that is the Shenandoah Valley.

 Great Views

		MILESTONES
►1	0.0	Riprap Hollow parking area
►2	0.9	Wildcat Ridge Trail leaves right
►3	1.4	Swimming hole
►4	1.7	Waterfalls
►5	2.8	Crest of Rocks Mountain
►6	3.0	View
►7	3.4	Chimney Rock

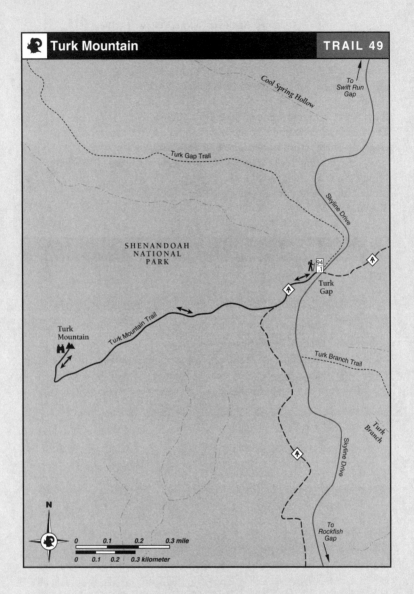

To
Swift Run
Gap

Cool Spring Hollow

Turk Gap Trail

Skyline Drive

SHENANDOAH
NATIONAL
PARK

94
1

Turk
Gap

Turk
Mountain

Turk Mountain Trail

Turk Branch Trail

Turk
Branch

Skyline Drive

N

0   0.1   0.2   0.3 mile

0   0.1   0.2   0.3 kilometer

To
Rockfish
Gap

Turk Mountain

This was my first hike ever at Shenandoah National Park. Turk Mountain makes a great initiation hike for park visitors entering Shenandoah from the southern end. But no matter where you come from, you will not be disappointed by the outstanding views from the mountain's rocky summit.

Best Time

Hikers come here for the views and the rock outcrops. Any time after cold fronts pass through or other clear days is good.

Finding the Trail

The Turk Gap parking area is located at milepost 94.1 on the east side of Skyline Drive, 10.5 miles north of the Rockfish Gap Entrance Station.

Trail Description

Start your hike at Turk Gap. ▶1 Cross Skyline Drive and begin descending on the Appalachian Trail (AT), southbound. Immediately enter a stand of pines. Be sure to take the trail to the left once you cross the road. The trail to the right is the Turk Gap Trail. Walk under mountain laurel, maple, and chestnut oaks. Arrive at a trail junction at 0.2 mile. ▶2 Veer right on the lesser-used Turk Mountain Trail, descending to an unnamed gap at 0.5 mile. ▶3 Turk Mountain rises through the trees.

The trail climbs the rocky east slope of Turk Mountain cloaked in hickory-oak forest and soon

TRAIL USE
Dayhiking

LENGTH
2.4 miles, 2–2½ hours

CUMULATIVE ELEVATION +/-
+500'/-500'

DIFFICULTY
− 1 **2** 3 4 5 +

TRAIL TYPE
Out & Back

START & FINISH
N38° 7.751'
W78° 47.089'

FEATURES
Ridgeline
Summit
Autumn Colors
Geologic Interest
Great Views
Secluded

FACILITIES
None

▲ Ridgeline

Autumn Colors

Geologic Interest

Summit

Great Views

Outstanding views
await from a
rocky summit.

enters a rock field. Continue through the rock field. The trail is rockier too.

The Turk Mountain Trail comes to a sharp right turn at 1.1 miles. ▶4 You can scramble onto the rocks to your left for southerly views, but the big boulders are unstable and the views are better atop the summit. The trail continues to the right, then passes among some large boulders just before attaining the crest of the mountain.

At the crest, turn right to walk an irregular rock ridge, pocked with short trees that have gained purchase on thin soils. And then you make it to an elevated rock outcrop and the summit of Turk Mountain (2,981 feet) at 1.2 miles. ▶5 The views are outstanding. Below, a talus slope lays bare the mountainside, opening westerly views into Crimora and the Shenandoah Valley below. To your north rises wave upon wave of wooded mountains. On the far side of the valley are the Allegheny Mountains and the George Washington National Forest. Back to the east is Middle Mountain with its radio towers. To the south stands Calf Mountain, which is also growing radio towers. The talus slope itself is an exquisite jumble of whitish-gray broken rocks, resembling play blocks of mountain giants, upon which no human walks.

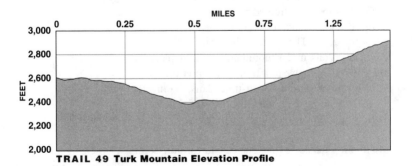

TRAIL 49 Turk Mountain Elevation Profile

FLORA

Indian Ghost Pipe

This rich slope is a great place to see an unusual plant, one of North America's strangest wildflowers, Indian ghost pipe. This white plant, with a flowerlike end, has no chlorophyll and resembles white clay pipes Cherokee Indians used for smoking tobacco. It can be seen in midsummer in Shenandoah. Ghost pipe obtains its nutrients from other plants, in a complex relationship with fungi that is not completely understood. Do not pick the ghost pipe—not that you would want it for a bouquet—because the ghost pipe's flesh soon blackens when cut or even bruised and oozes a clear, gelatinous substance. Its natural white color and tendency to "melt" after it has been picked also gives it the moniker "ice plant."

MILESTONES

▶1	0.0	Turk Gap parking area at milepost 94.1
▶2	0.2	Turk Mountain Trail leaves left from the AT
▶3	0.5	Gap
▶4	1.1	Right turn
▶5	1.2	Top of Turk Mountain with views

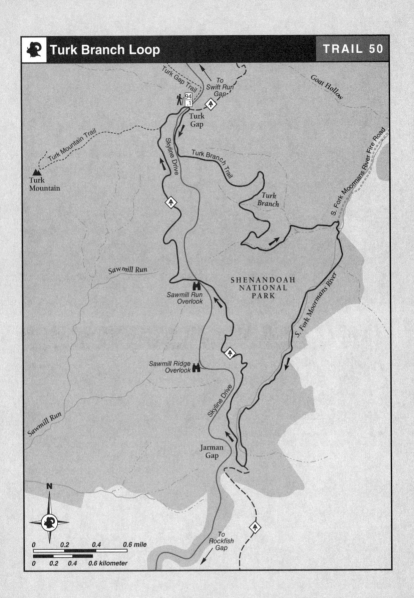

Turk Branch Loop

TRAIL 50

Turk Gap Trail

To Swift Run Gap

Goat Hollow

94

1

Turk Gap

Turk Mountain Trail

Turk Branch Trail

S. Fork Moormans River Fire Road

Turk Mountain

Skyline Drive

Turk Branch

Sawmill Run

SHENANDOAH NATIONAL PARK

S. Fork Moormans River

Sawmill Run Overlook

Sawmill Ridge Overlook

Sawmill Run

Skyline Drive

Jarman Gap

N

To Rockfish Gap

0   0.2   0.4   0.6 mile

0   0.2   0.4   0.6 kilometer

Turk Branch Loop

This loop traverses the park's most southerly and seemingly most forgotten reaches. Leave the crest of the Blue Ridge and descend along remote Turk Branch, passing old homesites where Turk Branch meets South Fork Moormans River. Head up the uppermost part of the rocky South Fork Moormans River Valley to meet the Appalachian Trail (AT). Hike north on Shenandoah's master path, gaining limited views amid the pines and oaks before returning to Turk Gap. Though the elevation change is nearly 1,200 feet, the trail grades are never sharp.

Best Time

This is a good hike when other trails are busy, such as during summer and on holiday weekends. In spring you can enjoy streamside wildflowers and better view the trailside homesites. In fall, autumn colors show. You will find solitude year-round beyond the AT.

Finding the Trail

The Turk Gap parking area is located at milepost 94.1 on Skyline Drive, 10.5 miles north of the Rockfish Gap Entrance Station, on the east side of the drive.

Trail Description

The hardest part of this loop may be finding its beginning. Look for the concrete signpost directly beside Skyline Drive leaving south from the Turk

TRAIL USE
Dayhiking, Backpacking
LENGTH
7.5 miles, 4–5 hours
CUMULATIVE ELEVATION +/-
-1,175'/+1,175'
DIFFICULTY
– 1 2 3 **4** 5 +
TRAIL TYPE
Loop
START & FINISH
N38° 7.751'
W78° 47.089'

FEATURES
Stream
Ridgeline
Autumn Colors
Wildflowers
Waterfall
Historic Interest
Secluded

FACILITIES
None

Gap parking area. ▶1 Do not take the unmarked trail leaving from the end of the parking area farthest from Skyline Drive. Make sure you are on the yellow-blazed Turk Branch Trail, and trace an old roadbed running parallel to Skyline Drive. Walk downhill through an oak-dominated forest. Skyline Drive rises to your right. At 0.3 mile, the Turk Branch Trail leads east, away from Skyline Drive. Descend on a dry ridgeline heavy with mountain laurel, scrub pines, and blueberries. Views of Bucks Elbow Mountain open between the trees.

Make a hard turn to the right at 1.0 mile. Descend to cross upper Turk Branch at 1.3 miles. ▶2 Black birch, maple, and cherry rise amid vines and ferns. Push over a rib ridge to cross a tributary of Turk Branch. Notice the stonework that has been done to level the old roadbed as it descends to cross Turk Branch again at 2.2 miles. ▶3 A low-flowing slab cascade drops above the Turk Branch crossing. Scant water keeps this fall modest and a lesser-visited destination.

Turk Branch valley widens. White pines shade the trailside flats. Piled stones, rock walls, and leveled land indicate a homesite to the left of the trail. Meet the South Fork Moormans River Fire Road at 2.5 miles. ▶4 A survey marker has been embedded into a boulder at the junction. Turn right here, and

▲ Ridgeline

🏞 Stream

🏔 Waterfall

🌼 Wildflowers

🧍 Secluded

TRAIL 50 Turk Branch Loop Elevation Profile

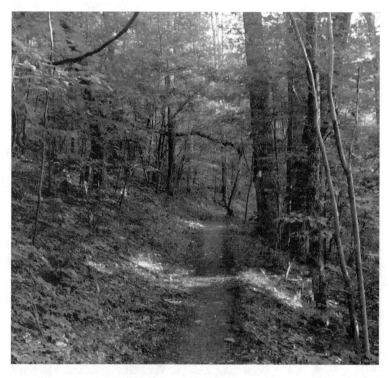

The Appalachian Trail *is a pleasant, level track in stretches*

rock-hop Turk Branch under sycamores aplenty. Ascend to soon step over South Fork Moormans River, which is but a small creek at this point. Watch for a few hemlocks that are hanging on. Pass a second homesite to the left of the trail, marked by rock walls, a clearing, a crumbling chimney, and metal relics. Please leave the remnants for others to discover and enjoy.

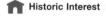 **Historic Interest**

The grade steepens as the hollow narrows beyond the homesite. At 3.1 miles, cross South Fork Moormans River, then bisect a natural gas–line clearing. Step over what's left of the river one more time, and then intersect the AT at 4.3 miles, just below

Ridgeline

Jarman Gap. ►5 Turn right here, hiking northbound on the AT. Dip along South Fork Moormans River one last time before ascending the east flank of the Blue Ridge, gaining views of Bucks Elbow Mountain across the Moormans River Valley. Climb more to cross the natural gas–line clearing at 5.0 miles. Top out on a piney knob at 5.4 miles. Windswept oaks and low-slung blueberries rise from the slaty soil. Views soon open to the south and west as the AT levels off. Sawmill Ridge and Turk Mountain stand in the distance.

Cross Skyline Drive and reach Sawmill Run Overlook at 6.0 miles. ►6 Begin climbing beyond Skyline Drive. Curve right past a side trail leading left through tangled woods to a spring. Level off, then undulate along the path lined with blueberry bushes, mountain laurel, and sassafras.

The latter deciduous tree can be found throughout the Old Dominion and here, along the AT. The AT along this stretch of the Blue Ridge makes for pleasant hiking without extensive elevation changes.

Intersect the Turk Mountain Trail at 7.3 miles. ►7 Keep north on the AT, and dip through some pines to emerge at Turk Gap at 7.5 miles and end your loop. ►8

Sassafras Trees

FLORA

Sassafras trees are easy to identify. Their leaves have three basic shapes: oval, three-lobed, and mitten-shaped. Mature sassafras trees have a reddish-brown, deeply furrowed bark. They are known for their aromatic scent. Scratch the bark away from a twig, and the sweet smell is unmistakable. American natives used sassafras for medicinal purposes. Pioneers and even people today make tea by boiling sassafras roots. Birds eat the berries. The wood of sassafras shrinks when dried and is used for fence posts and hand tools.

🚶 MILESTONES

▶1　0.0　Turk Gap parking area at milepost 94.1

▶2　1.3　Cross Turk Branch

▶3　2.2　Cross Turk Branch, and pass a cascade

▶4　2.5　Right on South Fork Moormans River Fire Road

▶5　4.3　Right on the AT

▶6　6.0　Cross Skyline Drive at Sawmill Run Overlook

▶7　7.3　Turk Mountain Trail leaves left

▶8　7.5　Turk Gap parking area at milepost 94.1

Local Resources

National Park Service

Shenandoah National Park
3655 US Highway 211 East
Luray, VA 22835
www.nps.gov/shen
General information: (540) 999-3500

The park's website has a wealth of information. They even have multimedia presentations about the park (**www.nps.gov/shen/photosmultimedia/index. htm**). If you can't find the information you desire on the website, then call the main park number and follow the prompts.

Other Area Resources

George Washington and Jefferson National Forests
5162 Valleypointe Parkway
Roanoke, VA 24019
www.fs.usda.gov/gwj
Supervisor's office: (888) 265-0019

Shenandoah visitors sometimes use the George Washington National Forest, which borders Shenandoah's south and west sides.

Shenandoah Valley Travel Association
PO Box 1040
New Market, VA 22844
www.visitshenandoah.org
(800) 847-4878

This website is your best portal to contact the tourist bureaus of the greater Shenandoah Valley from top to bottom. Simply find your geographic area of interest, click on the link for that area, and find your desired information.

Shenandoah Partnership Groups

Shenandoah National Park Association
3655 US Highway 211 East
Luray, VA 22835
www.snpbooks.org
(540) 999-3582

Established in 1950, the Shenandoah National Park Association (SNPA)
supports the interpretive and educational activities of Shenandoah
National Park. Since its inception, the SNPA has donated more than 2 mil-
lion dollars to the park through its sales of books, maps, merchandise, and
memorabilia. Check their website for a wealth of books and other sources
of information about your Shenandoah area of interest.

Potomac Appalachian Trail Club
118 Park Street SE
Vienna, VA 22180
www.patc.net
(703) 242-0968

The Potomac Appalachian Trail Club (PATC) is a large organization that
helps maintain the Appalachian Trail and other trails throughout much of
the Mid-Atlantic. They also maintain many trails within the Shenandoah
National Park trail system. Within the park they maintain backcountry cabins for rent. The PATC creates the primary trail maps used for Shenandoah's
three districts, which are sale online and at park visitor centers. Joining the
PATC is a great way to give your time, talent, and treasure to Shenandoah
National Park.

Index

A

animals of Shenandoah National
    Park, 5–6
Appalachian Trail (AT), 17, 33, 50,
    77, 101, 146, 185, 192, 201,
    225–226, 236
areas of region, xvii
Austin Mountain, 231–232
Austin Mountain and Madison Run
    Loop, 238, 282–287

B

Bear Church Rock from Bootens Gap,
    118, 200–203
Bear Church Rock via Staunton River,
    117, 196–199
Bearfence Mountain, 205
Bearfence Mountain Rock Scramble,
    110, 209, 210
best time (trail descriptor), xix
Big Branch Falls via Moormans River,
    239, 241–245, 305–308
Big Devils Stairs Vista, 22, 36–41
Big Run, 253
Big Run Loop, 237, 270–282
birds of Shenandoah National Park,
    5–6
Blackrock Loop, 238, 300–304
Bolen Cemetery, 59
Brown Mountain, 252–254
Browns Gap, 291
Browns Gap Turnpike, 277

C

Cedar Run Falls, 116, 168–173
cell phones, 11–12

Central District
    Bear Church Rock from Bootens
        Gap, 200–203
    Bear Church Rock via Staunton
        River, 196–199
    Cedar Run Falls, 168–173
    Corbin Cabin Hike, 134–137
    Falls of Whiteoak Canyon,
        162–167
    Hawksbill Summit, 174–177
    Hazel Country Loop, 130–133
    Hazel Falls and Cave, 126–129
    Hazeltop and Rapidan Camp
        Loop, 190–195
    Lewis Spring Falls Loop, 184–189
    map, 112
    Marys Rock via The Pinnacle,
        120–125
    Millers Head, 156–161
    Old Rag Loop, 138–143
    overview of, 109–111
    Pocosin Mission, 212–217
    Robertson Mountain, 150–155
    Rose River Falls Loop, 178–183
    Saddleback Mountain Loop,
        224–227
    South River Falls Loop, 218–224
    Stony Man Loop, 144–149
    trail features table, 113
    trail summaries, 114–119
    USGS topographic maps, 111
Chimney Rock, 239, 309–313
Chimney Rock via Riprap Hollow,
    239, 314–319
Civilian Conservation Corps
    (CCC), 160
clothing for hiking, 10

compass, and maps, 11
Compton Peak, 22, 32–35
Conway River Loop, 118, 204–210
copperhead snakes, 6
Corbin, George and Nee, 137
Corbin Cabin Hike, 115, 134–137

D

Dark Hollow Falls, 180
dayhiking, 3
Dickey Ridge Historic Hike, 22, 26–31
Dickey Ridge Visitor Center, 17, 27
difficulty (trail descriptor), xx, xxii
Doyles River, 290–292
drinking water, 10–11
Dundo Picnic Area, Loft Mountain, 231

E

elevation (trail descriptor), xx–xxi, xxii
Elkwallow Loop, 24, 76–81
equipment, hiking, 10–12
etiquette, trail, 12–13

F

Falls Loop from Browns Gap, 238,
    288–293
Falls of Whiteoak Canyon, 116,
    162–167
features (trail descriptor), xx
fish of Shenandoah National Park, 6
flora of Shenandoah National Park,
    4–5
food, 11
Fraser fir, 176
Furnace Mountain via Blacktop, 238,
    294–299

G

gear, hiking, 10–12
geography of Shenandoah National
    Park, 3–4
George Washington National Forest,
    330

Giardia parasite, 11
GPS (Global Positioning System)
    receiver, handheld, 11
gypsy moths, 297

H

handheld GPS receivers, 11
Hawksbill Summit, 110, 116, 161,
    174–177
Hazel Country Loop, 114, 130–133
Hazel Falls and Cave, 114, 126–129
Hazeltop and Rapidan Camp Loop,
    117, 190–195
Heiskell Hollow Loop, 24, 72–75
Hightop, 236
hiking
    clothing, 10
    drinking water, 10–11
    food, maps, cell phones, 11–12
    gear, 12
    preparing, planning, 9–10
    trail etiquette, 12–13
Hogsback Mountain, 43, 45, 49
Hoover, Herbert, 194
horseback riders, 13
Howard, William H., 290
Hughes River, 135, 137

I

Indian ghost pipe plant, 323

J

Jackson, Gen. Stonewall, 291
Jefferson National Forest, 330
Jeremys Run Loop
    Knob Mountain, 25, 88–93
    Neighbor Mountain, 25, 94–99
Jones Mountain, 201, 203

K

Keyser Run, 55, 56–57, 58
Knob Mountain, Jeremys Run Loop,
    25, 88–93

L

legend, map, xxi
Lewis Spring Falls Loop, 117,
    184–189
litter, 12
Little Devils Stairs Loop, 23, 54–59
local resources, 330–331
Loft Mountain Loop, 237, 258–263
loop hikes, 3
Lower Whiteoak Falls, 165

M

map legend, xxi
maps. *See also specific trails*
    Central District, 111, 112
    essential, 11
    North District, 19, 20
    Shenandoah overview, vi–vii
    South District, 233, 234
    USGS topographic (list), 19,
        111, 233
Marys Rock via The Pinnacle, 114,
    120–125
Mathews Arm Campground, 18, 49,
    67, 73, 77, 83
Millers Head, 116, 156–161
Moormans River, 305–307

N

National Park Service, 330
navigation, 13
Neighbor Mountain, 92
Neighbor Mountain, Jeremys Run
    Loop, 25, 94–99
Nichols, Harvey, 199
North District
    Big Devils Stairs Vista, 22, 36–41
    Compton Peak, 22, 32–35
    Dickey Ridge Historic Hike, 22,
        26–31
    Elkwallow Loop, 24, 76–81
    Heiskell Hollow Loop, 24, 72–75

Knob Mountain, Jeremys Run
    Loop, 88–93
Little Devils Stairs Loop, 23,
    54–59
map, 20
Neighbor Mountain, Jeremys Run
    Loop, 94–99
Overall Run Falls, 23, 48–53
Overall Run Loop, 24, 66–71
overview of, 17–19
Piney River Falls, 24, 82–87
Sugarloaf Loop, 23, 42–47
Thornton River Loop, 100–105
Traces Nature Trail, 23, 60–65
trail features table, 21
trail summaries, 22–25
trails, 15
USGS topographic maps, 19
North Fork Moormans River, 305

O

Old Rag Loop, 115, 138–143
old-growth forests, 216
Overall Run Falls, 23, 48–53
Overall Run Loop, 24, 66–71

P

Patterson Ridge Loop, 237, 264–269
permits
    Central District, 111
    North District, 19
    South District, 233
pets, 8
Piney River Falls, 24, 82–87
plants of Shenandoah National Park,
    4–5
Pocosin Mission, 111, 118, 212–217
Pollock, George Freeman, 152, 157–
    158, 160
Potomac Appalachian Trail Club
    (PATC), 214, 227, 331

R

Rapidan River, 198
Rapidan Wildlife Management Area, 106, 110, 202, 205, 221
ratings, difficulty, xxii
rattlesnakes, 6
red spruce, 176
regional map, xvi
resources, local, 330–331
Robertson Mountain, 115, 150–155
Rocks Mountain, 318
Rocky Mount Loop, 231, 236, 246–251
Rocky Mountain Loop, 231, 236, 252–257
Rockytop and Big Run Loop, 237, 276–281
Rockytop Mountain, 231
Roosevelt, Franklin Delano, 160
Rose River Falls Loop, 178–183
Rose River Falls Loop, 117

S

Saddleback Mountain Loop, 119, 224–227
sassafras trees, 328
seasons, 7
shagbark hickories, 256
Shenandoah National Park
    introduction to, 1–8
    map, vi–vii
    trails (tables), viii–xi
    when to visit, 6–7
Shenandoah National Park Association, 331
Shenandoah Valley Travel Association, 330
Skyland Resort, 157–158
Smith Run Fire of 2011, 1, 33
South District
    Austin Mountain and Madison Run Loop, 238, 282–287

Big Branch Falls via Moormans River, 239, 241–245, 305–308
Big Run Loop, 237, 270–282
Blackrock Loop, 238, 300–304
Chimney Rock, 239, 309–313
Chimney Rock via Riprap Hollow, 239, 314–319
Falls Loop from Browns Gap, 238, 288–293
Furnace Mountain via Blacktop, 238, 294–299
Hightop, 236
Loft Mountain Loop, 237, 258–263
map, 234
overview of, 231–233
Patterson Ridge Loop, 237, 264–269
Rocky Mount Loop, 236, 246–251
Rocky Mountain Loop, 236, 252–257
Rockytop and Big Run Loop, 237, 276–281
trail features table, 235
trail summaries, 236–240
Turk Branch Loop, 240, 324–329
Turk Mountain, 240, 320–323
USGS topographic maps, 233
South Fork Moormans River, 327–328
South River Falls Loop, 118, 218–224
Staunton River, 197–199
Stony Man Loop, 115, 144–149
striped maples ("moosewood"), 128
Sugarloaf Loop, 23, 42–47

T

temperature, monthly averages (table), 7
Thornton River Loop, 100–105
timber rattlesnakes, 6

Top Trails
    organization of, xvi–xviii
    series, v
topography of Shenandoah National
    Park, 3–4
Traces Nature Trail, 23, 60–65
trail etiquette, 12–13
trails
    Central District summaries,
      114–119
    choosing, xix–xx
    navigating entries, xviii
    North District summaries, 22–25
    selection of, 8
    Shenandoah National Park
      (tables), viii–xi
    South District summaries,
      236–240
Trayfoot Mountain, 296, 297–298,
    312

Turk Branch Loop, 240, 324–329
Turk Mountain, 232, 240, 320–323

U

USGS topographic maps
    Central District (list), 111
    North District (list), 19
    South District (list), 233

W

water, drinking, 10–11
weather, 7
websites, local resources, 330–331
woolly adelgid, 290–291

Y

yellow birches, 222